A Diary of Gastric Bypass Surgery

A Diary of Gastric Bypass Surgery

WHEN THE BENEFITS OUTWEIGH THE COSTS

Darlene K. Drummond

STATE UNIVERSITY OF NEW YORK PRESS

Published by
State University of New York Press, Albany

© 2008 State University of New York

For information, contact State University of New York Press, Albany, NY
www.sunypress.edu

Production by Marilyn P. Semerad
Marketing by Susan M. Petrie

Library of Congress Cataloging in Publication Data

Drummond, Darlene K., 1959–
A diary of gastric bypass surgery : when the benefits outweigh the
costs / Darlene K. Drummond.
    p. cm.
Includes bibliographical references and index.
ISBN 978-0-7914-7439-6 (hardcover : alk. paper)
ISBN 978-0-7914-7440-2 (pbk. : alk. paper) 1. Drummond, Darlene K.,
1959—Health. 2. Gastric bypass—Patients—Biography. I. Title.
RD540.5.D78 2008
362.197'5530092—dc22
[B]

                                        2007033699

10 9 8 7 6 5 4 3 2 1

*This story is dedicated to the memory of
Francenia McLean Chandler,
my mother,
who in life taught me the value of a good education,
and in death . . . compassion.*

Contents

Preface

The following is a narrative, a personal account of my experience with weight-loss surgery based on the journal I kept from 2002 through 2006. Even though this story does not take the form of traditional scholarship in reporting generalizable conclusions from so-called empirical evidence, it is scholarship.

My purpose in presenting you with this autoethnography (see Ellis & Bochner, 2000, for more about this form of scholarship) is not to make staunch claims about weight-loss surgery, health, or communication; it is simply to invite you to relive and share with me one specific point in time in my lived experience. The story, presented to you in the tradition of phenomenology (see Crotty, 1998), is a careful and very raw description of my everyday lived experiences, including my perceptions, beliefs, memories, decisions, feelings, judgments, evaluations, and physical activities as they actually occurred.

Admittedly, my approach is even different from that of traditional autoethnography—purposely. I do not interrupt the telling of my story by weaving into it scholarly or intellectual interpretations and analyses grounded in social scientific reports. However, at the end of each chapter I suggest a few readings and theoretical frameworks that would be appropriate for discussing the events that occurred. These suggestions are limited, allowing the reader, whether scholar or layperson, to make his or her own decisions on how to frame particular events. In my attempt to bridge personal narrative with scholarly inquiry, my primary goal is to make the *story,* not my analyses, as accessible to as many readers as possible. Therefore, the knowledge and insight *you* as an individual might provide in understanding what I have experienced is privileged and expected. For me, knowledge is personal, always temporal and contextual.

As Bochner (1994, p. 33) states, and I agree, "The power of autobiographical stories often rests on the degree to which they perform the dual function of being sufficiently unique to evoke comparisons and sufficiently universal to elicit identification." My experience is unique in that it represents a very specific standpoint (Collins, 1991), that of an African American woman coping with chronic illness who has weight-loss surgery. But under no circumstances am I suggesting my experience is representative of all African American women who have had the surgery (see Bell, Orbe, Drummond, & Camara, 2000). Ultimately, I am a human being like you with a multiplicity of identities that are constantly evolving; and I defy anyone, regardless of race, gender, or social class to fail to see themselves in these pages.

My story presents human experience as multilayered, highly impacted by issues of race, gender, and social class, but, most important, it focuses on the conversations we have with one another. This book is for the academic or health professional who is looking for a novel way to teach or talk about health experiences. But it is also for the ordinary person living with, or who knows someone living with, a chronic illness like diabetes, high blood pressure, or obesity.

I have used the real names of my family members, friends, and co-workers in recognition of their past and continuing support. However, the names of all health professionals who are not related to me have been changed.

REFERENCES

Bell, K. E., Orbe, M. P., Drummond, D. K., & Camara, S. K. (2000). Accepting the challenge of centralizing without essentializing: Black feminist thought and African American women's communicative experiences. *Women's Studies in Communication, 23*(1), 41–62.

Bochner, A. P. (1994). Perspectives on inquiry II: Theories and stories. In M. L. Knapp & G. R. Miller (Eds.), *Handbook of Interpersonal Communication* (2nd ed., pp. 21–41). Thousand Oaks: Sage.

Collins, P. H. (1991). *Black Feminist Thought*. New York: Routledge.

Crotty, M. (1998). *The Foundations of Social Research*. London: Sage.

Ellis, C., & Bochner, A. P. (2000). Autoethnography, personal narrative, reflexivity: Researcher as subject. In N. K. Denzin & Y. S. Lincoln (Eds.), *Handbook of Qualitative Research* (2nd ed.). Thousand Oaks, CA: Sage.

1

Inheritance

January 11, 2002

Standing beside her hospital bed, I slowly reached for the small warm hands that have gently brushed my face in love for years and tapped my back in support at each of my individual triumphs—high school graduation, college graduation, my dissertation defense, and the job that brought me home again to North Carolina. I smiled to myself as I remembered the numerous times these fingers playfully pointed at me in a side-to-side motion accompanied by uplifted eyebrows and a slight frown indicating disappointment at the stupid things that frequently came out of my mouth.

My mother has beautiful strong hands—slender fingers with long natural nails, manicured and polished—a ring containing her children's birthstones on her left hand, and a thin silver watch on her wrist.

But today is different. Today the hands I hold are frail with short nails and chipped polish. The watch and ring are missing. Things have changed. My mother lay dead in a hospital bed. The complications of diabetes, high blood pressure, undiagnosed liver problems, and kidney failure had murdered her and robbed me of the love of my life. As I placed her hands on her chest, sadness and anger welled up inside me, and I left the room in silence, as her guardians, my sister, brother and sister-in-law remained.

In our grief, each of us struggled to move on with our lives. Throughout the following months, I was haunted by long-lost memories of disease and illness run amok in my family and the lessons I failed to understand. My mother was not the first in our family to suffer from the complications of diabetes and high blood pressure. Diabetes and hypertension had become the norm. The two were so much ingrained within the fabric of our lives that they became invisible to our conscious minds. But my grief drove one fact clearly to the forefront of my mind—nearly every adult member of my family over 35 has diabetes or hypertension or both, including my sister, brother, father, aunts, and uncles.

I had to know. Did I have diabetes? Did I have hypertension? Were my persistent infections, dry skin, gum disease, blurring vision, and weight gain significant? Would my next 20 years be filled with kidney dialysis, heart disease, stroke, and gangrene? Would my experience be different from every other adult in my family? I had to know.

Diagnoses

SEPTEMBER 13, 2002. I went to the Mallard Creek Family Practice to see May Land, my family doctor, for my annual physical. I told her I had been under enormous stress in trying to deal with the death of my mother due to complications of diabetes, hypertension, and kidney failure. As the executrix of her estate, I felt pressured to handle everything perfectly to prevent dissension in my family. I was depressed but felt there might be something else wrong with me. With water retention in my legs, excessive thirst, and constant fatigue, I just did not feel well. On some level I knew I was diabetic. What I sought was confirmation.

"Can you give me a test to determine whether or not I am diabetic?" I asked.

"Let's just do a routine physical with pap smear," Dr. Land said. "You haven't had a pap smear in over two years. Let's get that done today. Okay?"

Annoyed, I repeated that I was interested in finding out if I had diabetes. I confided I had not had a sexual relationship in years and seriously doubted my problems stemmed from my vaginal area. Dr. Land stated I would have to have a three-hour glucose test. "The test is very expensive," she said. "We couldn't do it today because you are required to fast before taking it. You would need to abstain from eating or drinking anything for 24 hours before the test."

"I can do that. Can we schedule it for this week? We can do the physical today except for the pap smear. I will do that later because I need to know as soon as possible if I have diabetes."

Sighing, Dr. Land agreed, proceeded with the physical, reiterated the importance of a pap smear and told me to arrange for the glucose test at the checkout window.

The next day I arrived at the doctor's office before 8:00 a.m. A nurse took and recorded my blood pressure and tested my blood sugar. My blood pressure was moderately high at 130/76 and blood sugar 135. The nurse stated that if normal my blood sugar should not be higher than 110. She instructed me to sit in the waiting area until it was time to record the second series of numbers. As I sat quietly, I watched other patients and used the time to grade papers and prepare lecture notes.

After an hour, my blood sugar was tested again. It had risen to 257. I knew from the frown on the nurse's face that this was bad news. Alone and once again in the waiting room, I prayed for my glucose level to drop. After another hour passed, the nurse tested my blood glucose again and it had dropped slightly to 240. I was happy to hear this until the nurse said it should be 140 or below. Dejected, I agonized that I indeed was what I dreaded more than anything—diabetic.

Grading papers and reading did not distract me from this fear. All I could see was my mother's face pleading with me to take care of myself. I cried, brokenhearted. How could I let this happen? Several doctors had warned me of this eventuality if I did not get my weight under control. I knew the havoc diabetes had wreaked with my family. I had witnessed the long suffering of my beloved mother and still had not heeded her warnings to make health my priority. Instead I spent a great deal of time and energy rationalizing that I led a healthy lifestyle. I exercised—not *regularly,* but I did exercise. I ate healthy foods—most of the time.

No, I did not. I did not exercise regularly. I did not exercise semi-regularly. Every blue moon is a more accurate characterization of how often I exercised. Ate healthy foods? Only if eating fast foods nearly every day, two to three times a day and steak and fried potatoes every Friday counted as healthy. For the first time, I was honest with myself. I had *not* done what I needed to do to achieve and maintain good health.

The final hour passed and my blood sugar was tested again. It had dropped 20 points to 220—only 20 points lower than the previous reading. Dr. May Land confirmed what I now knew.

"You have diabetes and your blood pressure is too high," she said. "With the diabetes you need to be concerned with your blood pressure level, too."

"Am I hypertensive?"

"Your blood pressure is higher than it should be," she said. "We need to keep an eye on it."

The family curse had befallen me.

Dr. Land handed me three prescriptions—Glucotrol, Glucophague, and Diovan. She explained that the first two drugs were designed to control my diabetes while the third was an anti-hypertension drug. In addition, I was given a prescription for a Glucometer to test my blood sugar at least three times a day every day. And I was instructed to attend a diabetes education class in downtown Charlotte, which I found ironic because I thought there was nothing a class could teach me that I had not already learned firsthand.

Then, hesitantly, Dr. Land mentioned that I might want to consider gastric bypass surgery. "A few of my patients have had great success with the procedure, and you may be a good candidate," she said. "Dr. Bozeman of Concord, North Carolina, comes highly recommended." She instructed me to see if her assistant could arrange a consultation for me to learn more about the procedure. The office assistant said Dr. Rode Bozeman had a waiting list and I would probably not be able to get an appointment for six months. She suggested I try to get his attention through his Web site. At the checkout window, I paid my $15 co-payment and noted the $287 balance owed.

I headed to the drugstore to fill my prescriptions. Even with health insurance I was out-of-pocket $123.32 for a month's supply of drugs. I sat in my car for nearly 20 minutes crying before I felt strong enough and alert enough to drive myself home. I was mentally exhausted, fearful, and angry. How could I possibly endure years of coping with diabetes and hypertension? How could someone who hated taking aspirin deal with taking three medications a day! I had always suffered through the common cold because of my fear of medications and now I was told that my survival depended on taking these medications on a regular basis. Damn, damn, *damn*! I feared the long-term consequences that I instinctively knew would occur if I took these drugs for years. My mother had taken similar medications for more than 15 years and, even though no doctor had said so, I believed that the long-term use of them aided in the failure of her kidneys and liver. Would this happen to me, too?

I have read many books and academic journal articles on the subject of diabetes, and knew that Americans died of complications of diabetes and hypertension at alarming rates, and African Americans died at even more alarming rates. Nevertheless, I was afraid at the thought of going to a diabetes education class and meeting more people with diabetes. I did not want to meet another African American with diabetes and hear about another African American starting kidney dialysis.

Getting a Consultation

To get a consultation with Dr. Rode Bozeman, one must first visit his Web site and fill out a patient information form via the Internet. The site discusses the process for getting a meeting with the surgeon, requirements for surgery, how laparoscopic gastric bypass is performed, and the risks and benefits of the surgery. The patient information form is comprehensive, requesting personal identification information such as insurance, employment, gender, and race. The patient is required to disclose weight information and detail all diets partaken and exercise programs attempted. Questions address counseling experiences, medications taken, and the history of obesity and other serious illnesses in one's family. The majority of the questions ask the patient to evaluate his or her current health situation by asking whether he or she has experienced a variety of ailments or diseases such as shortness of breath, diabetes, sleep apnea, lung disease, asthma, thyroid disease, high blood pressure, heart disease, high cholesterol, incontinence, gall bladder disease, and kidney disease.

It took me a couple of days to complete the form because I had to look up addresses and medical information from a variety of sources. I keep health-related paperwork, especially lab reports, receipts from office visits, and notices from my health insurance company. Admittedly, my files are not well-organized. Nevertheless, this practice of never throwing anything away paid off, making it easier to complete the patient information form to get a consultation.

As I waited for word from Dr. Bozeman's office, my sister Marlene, a registered nurse at Frye Regional Medical Center in Hickory, North Carolina, sent me information on their surgical weight loss program. The packet contained a small booklet entitled "The Facts about Weight Loss Surgery," published by Ethicon Endo-Surgery, Inc., a Johnson & Johnson Company, and a video on the surgical procedure with patients discussing how it saved their lives. This was the first instructive information I read. It explained the differences between the various types of surgical weight-loss procedures and, as every other document, Web site, or book I referred to, touted the gastric bypass or "Roux-En-Y" as being the most effective. All the information I obtained about gastric bypass was from hospitals and surgeons specializing in this technique. I avoided nonmedical or nongovernment-sponsored health Web sites. The more useful and trustworthy sites included www.weight-losssurgeryinfo.com, the American Society for Bariatric Surgery's Web site at www.asbs.org, and the National Institutes of Health Web site www.nih.gov.

DISCUSSION QUESTIONS

1. How much do you know about your family's medical history? How relevant is this history in making decisions about your health care?

2. Do you feel comfortable talking about death and dying? Why or why not? How do Americans and other cultures view death and the process of dying?

3. How do you find out about various treatment options? Has a doctor ever suggested a treatment that surprised you? If so, what and why?

4. Have you ever been scared into changing your behavior? Explain what happened.

5. What racial differences exist in the diagnoses and lived experiences of individuals with chronic illnesses? If such differences exist, should we talk about them? If so, how?

SUGGESTED READINGS

Golin, C., DiMatteo, M. R., Duan, N., Leake, B., & Gelberg, L. (2002). Impoverished diabetic patients whose doctors facilitate their participation in medical decision making are more satisfied with their care. *Journal of General Internal Medicine, 17*, 866–875.

Hofmann, J. C., Wenger, N. S., David, R. B., Teno, J., Connors, A. F., Desbiens, N., Lynn, J., & Phillips, R. S. (1997). Patient preferences for communication with physicians about end-of-life decisions. *Annals of Internal Medicine, 127*, 1–12.

Maynard, D. W. (2004). On predicting a diagnosis as an attribute of a person. *Discourse Studies, 6*(1), 53–76.

Pudlinski, C. (2005). Doing empathy and sympathy: Caring responses to troubles tellings on a peer support line. *Discourse Studies, 7*(3), 267–288.

Wilkin, H. A., Ball-Rokeach, S. J. (2006). Reaching at risk groups: The importance of health storytelling in Los Angeles Latino media. *Journalism, 7*(3), 299–320.

2

Preoperative Evaluation

My First Meeting with the Bariatric Surgeon

DECEMBER 9, 2002. I awoke to the splash of rain against my bedroom sliding doors. Excited, I jumped out of bed, checked the alarm clock and dashed into the bathroom to wash and dress. I chose a loose-fitting green turtleneck sweater and blue jeans that were easy to get on and off, combed my hair, and decided to go makeup free. After checking myself in the mirror, I grabbed my wallet and an umbrella, and walked out of my front door headed for the parking lot.

My car was encased in melting ice. I fumbled with the car keys and tried to unlock the driver side door then felt the umbrella slip from my hands. When the door opened, I sat down, grabbed the umbrella from the ground and threw it on the passenger's seat. Rarely do I make it into the car without getting wet. I was irritated and began to wonder if I had made the right decision to see a bariatric surgeon. If it was meant to be, I told myself, I would make it to my appointment on time. If not, the rain, ice, and my mood would prevent my timely arrival and condemn me to a life of habitual fad dieting. Was this fear, or was I trying to prepare myself for possible disappointment if the doctor said I did not meet the requirements for surgery?

I drove north for nearly 20 minutes up I-85 to exit 60, Dale Earnhardt and Copperfield Drive to the Piedmont Surgical Clinic in Concord, North Carolina, for my 7:30 a.m. appointment, and arrived early—15 minutes early. It *was* meant to be. At least I was meant to meet and speak with this surgeon.

The clinic was not what I expected. It was a large, light-blue wood-framed building nestled among trees on the left-hand side of the road across from the entrance to the hospital. I had expected to see a modern, red-brick building with clean lines and hoped the dingy old building did not reflect the age or attitude of the doctor. I obeyed the signs to park in the back and entered the rear of the building, which opened into a large waiting room. I saw uphol-stered chairs, a water fountain, and bulletin boards covered with health information; in a separate area a group of nurses and a receptionist talked quietly behind a glass partition. As I walked around the room, the words "dry mouth" attracted my attention on one of the bulletin boards. Dry mouth . . . yes, I can relate. When I was diagnosed with diabetes and hypertension, my family doctor prescribed medications that caused dry mouth, and with braces on my teeth, the problem worsened. I was constantly looking for new ways to relieve the discomfort. The advertisement on the board endorsed a prescription medication for control of dry mouth, but I preferred to continue with mouth rinses than consider another prescription drug.

Two individuals, a middle-aged white woman weighing between 500 and 600 pounds and a young white man weighing between 400 and 500 pounds, sat in the waiting room. Both watched as I approached the receptionist. I wondered if they sus-pected why I was there, and I thought I spotted envy in their eyes. You know the look, the one that has that blaring question stated with direct eye contact, asking, "What the hell are you here for? What do you want?" Yes, I have used it quite a few times myself. But was I getting the look because I was obviously 200 to 300 pounds lighter? I rolled my eyes in self-defense and thought that I had as much right to be there as they did. For all they knew I could

be there for any number of reasons. Yeah, right. The man is a specialist in bariatric surgery! There is only one reason to see *him*!

All kinds of thoughts ran through my head as I tried to project a confident unfazed front: What's wrong with you? Why are you judging these people? Get a grip on yourself! Not everyone is interested in you! They do not care why you are here! Do you really care what they think? Hell *yeah*! Hell *no*!

But, no matter what I thought . . . I felt exposed . . . exposed as an individual who was admitting to being fat . . . too fat.

At the receptionist area was a sign indicating co-payment was due before seeing the doctor. I signed the sign-in sheet and the receptionist immediately requested the $255 fee for a new patient gastric bypass patient consultation. I wrote out the check and gave her my health insurance card and driver's license. She made a copy of the license and insurance card and returned them to me with a receipt. I sat down across from the severely obese female and waited.

Susan, who was in a wheelchair, introduced herself and asked if I was there to get information about gastric-bypass surgery. She excitedly informed me that her surgery was scheduled for the following week, but she also complained that the process had taken six months. I was shocked and thought six months is a long time! I hope it doesn't take that long for me! I might change my mind! Nevertheless, she had my attention and I eagerly listened as she shared with me why she was having the surgery. Susan admitted that her knees hurt constantly and that she could not walk a block without becoming winded. She believed the surgery would change her life for the better. I could see the hope and anticipation in her eyes. Before Susan could say anything else, her name was called and she wished me well and wheeled herself out of the receptionist area. I quietly thanked God that I could carry my own body weight without the need of a wheelchair. I thanked God that my weight had not reached 300 pounds and asked for forgiveness for wondering how anyone could allow themselves to get in such a physical state. *There but for the grace of God, go I . . .*

I waited 20 minutes before my name was called. Then a hurried nurse escorted me to a scale to take my weight (244 lbs) and height (5 ft 3½ in.). She neither bothered to engage in small talk nor look at me. She led me into a small room with a round table and a small television resting on a stand; here I would have to watch a 45-minute tape about the laparoscopic gastric bypass procedure before I could speak with the doctor. As I waited for the tape to begin, the young white man who had been in the waiting room joined me.

We introduced ourselves. Tom said he was considering the surgery because diabetes ran in his family and he was afraid to be the next one diagnosed. At 35 years of age he felt it inevitable due to his weight. He admitted he was afraid of the idea of surgery and did not know whether or not he would or could go through with the procedure. I did not comment, and together we watched the amateur video narrated by the bariatric surgeon, Dr. Rode Bozeman.

As the tape progressed, Tom squirmed and fidgeted with his pencil. I tried to suppress a smile as the sweat ran down his face, looked directly at him and asked if he was okay. I admit to a mild sense of pleasure from watching his discomfort in the midst of my unflinching composure. If Tom could not handle a video of the procedure, I, too, doubted he was ready to have the procedure done. *Damn, why do we get such pleasure out of other people's discomfort? What kind of person am I?* I reassured myself that I was a good person and was only reacting to his inability to handle gore. After all, I consider myself a connoisseur of horror, especially vampire movies.

The video was awful. If designing a video was a requirement for successfully completing medical school, Dr. Bozeman would not be practicing medicine. However informative, it was boring and failed to hold my attention. It was much too long. Dr. Bozeman was a monotone narrator, and the tape needed better graphics and better background music. One of the drawbacks of being a communication professor is the tendency to critique and possibly overanalyze every form of media and communication interaction

you observe. I reminded myself that my decision to have gastric bypass surgery should be and would be based on my assessment of Dr. Bozeman's medical abilities, not his video production.

As the video ended, Tom said, "I don't think I can go through with it!"

The nurse walked in and said the doctor was ready to see us. He would see me first. Tom and I got up from the table and left the room. As we walked down the hall, Tom told the nurse that he did not want to see the doctor, and he headed for the waiting area. I did not see him again.

The nurse took me to an examination room where I sat in a chair next to the examination table. Dr. Bozeman entered, introduced himself and sat on the other side of the examination table directly across from me. Blond, tall, and in excellent shape, he appeared to be 40-something. Not a man to waste time, he got straight to the point. As he reviewed my paperwork, he asked about the diets I had tried, who referred me to him, whether I understood the video, and whether I had any questions about the process. He seemed hurried, and I felt rushed.

The nurse took my blood pressure and asked me about my employment and the medications I was taking. She said I should meet with the scheduler after meeting with the doctor to have all the required tests arranged. When the nurse left, Dr. Bozeman explained to me that at a height of 5 ft 3½ in. and 244 pounds that I had a body mass index (BMI) of 44. He explained that my weight and various co-morbidities associated with obesity, including diabetes, hypertension, possible gastric reflux disease, and sleep apnea suggested that I might be a good candidate for the surgery. He quickly enumerated the various preoperative procedures I would have to endure for a proper evaluation to be done to determine if and when I could have the surgery. I was required to have electrocardiograms, psychological evaluations, X-rays of my chest to examine my gastrointestinal tract, and blood tests to evaluate my liver and kidney functioning. He handed me a stack of papers,

including a consent form, and told me to read the material thoroughly during the next few weeks and to contact him if I had any questions. We stood, shook hands, said it was nice to meet each other, and he was gone. I spent less than 10 minutes with him. Even though this made me feel a little uneasy, I was anxious to see the scheduler and get things under way. Clearly, Dr. Bozeman did not like to invest much time in potential clients until he had information confirming eligibility for surgery through the established preoperative procedures. I did not blame him.

Back in the front office area, Robin, the office manager and surgery scheduler, reiterated that I had to go through a series of required tests before the doctor would consider operating on me. I had the option of going with their established network of psychologists, endocrinologists, and nutritionists or choosing my own specialists. To simplify things I chose to go with their team. If they were networked, then they probably spent more time talking with each other and there would be less of the chance for miscommunication. I reasoned that the process would take less time and I would be better off with professionals who had already had extensive experience with bariatric patients and with one another. Plus, I did not want to deal with the added stress of running to and fro between the various clinics and hospitals in the metropolitan area to meet with and select my own specialists.

Our conversation turned to health insurance. Robin immediately reassured me that my health insurance carrier, the State of North Carolina Teachers' and State Employees' Comprehensive Major Medical Plan, would pay for the surgery. She would submit all of the necessary paperwork to get the process rolling and all I needed to do was follow through with my preoperative appointments. Robin scheduled my first series of tests, an upper G.I. series and an H-Pylori blood test for December 13, 2002. Then she set an appointment with a psychologist at the Northeast Psychological Group for Friday, January 17; an appointment with an endocrinologist for Wednesday, February 12, 2003 at 8:00 a.m. at

the NEMC Medical Arts Building; and an appointment with a nutritionist for Wednesday, February 12, 2003 at 10:00 a.m. at the Diabetes Management Center. All of the facilities were within 5 minutes of one another in Concord.

When I finally left the clinic, it was 9:45 a.m. I had spent more than two hours there and it was worth the time. Exuberant, I returned home and read all the literature given me. A couple of days later I received a card from Dr. Bozeman that stated, "You're important to us. Welcome to our practice and thank you for your confidence in us." That was a nice touch.

Completing the Required Diagnostic Tests

The Radiology Department of Northeast Medical Center is impressive. I approached the receptionist area, gave my name, and was handed a gadget that vibrated to inform me when to go through the door on my right for testing. The receptionist said the device was designed to protect the privacy of patients. They no longer call out names.

Before I had a chance to choose a magazine, the gadget vibrated and I was escorted by a nurse through the door to a dressing room. She instructed me to remove all my clothing and jewelry from the waist up and to put on a gown. I fumbled with the gown, trying to decide whether to tie it in the back or front. I tied it in the back.

An X-ray technician led me into a room where I was given a thick, nasty, extremely sweet drink called barium. Once the required ounces were consumed, the Upper G.I. Series began. Pictures were taken of my esophagus, stomach, and intestine. A doctor and the X-ray technician looked intently at the pictures. The doctor, who had not introduced himself, commented that I apparently had gastric reflux disease. He could see fluid rise up my esophagus and stand in my throat. He talked about how slow the

fluid moved through my system and informed me that the information would be relayed to my surgeon.

Then the X-ray technician led me back to the dressing room and handed me a form entitled "Northeast Medical Center Radiology Department Outpatient Discharge Instructions." Six different categories were listed on the form, with the first, "post barium studies," checked. The instructions beneath the label indicated that I could resume normal activities, should drink plenty of fluids throughout the day, including six 8-ounce glasses of water, and take a laxative if needed. "Drink as much water as you can today and you will feel fine," she said. "Sign the bottom and follow the signs to the lab."

I signed the form and handed it back to the technician. She gave me a copy and I crossed the hallway to the laboratory. Within 5 minutes, blood was drawn from my right arm and I was on my way back home. I smiled to myself as I realized I was one more step closer to my goal.

Health Insurance Authorization

The State of North Carolina Teachers' and State Employees' Comprehensive Major Medical Plan authorized surgery. I sent a copy of the authorization notice to the Piedmont Surgical Clinic, my surgeon's office. The notice signed by Hilda Jones, a medical review analyst, contained my name, Social Security number, date of birth, an authorization number, and a reference number. It indicated that a "Y-ST Surgical Procedure, GAST RESTRICT W/BYP-MORBID OBES; SHORT ROUX-EN-Y, 1 Unit was authorized for 1/8/03 – 3/9/03." Ms. Jones further advised, "This authorization is valid only for the dates listed above. Any continued length of stay or continuation of service will require you to submit a request for extension. This authorization is not valid and will not guarantee payment if (1) at the time the service is received, the benefits have

been exhausted or (2) at the time the services are received, there is no coverage."

Since it was already December and I had not completed all of the required preoperative evaluation stages, I knew that the clinic would have to ask for an extension. Nevertheless, I was satisfied with the way my insurance company and surgeon's office handled things.

Psychological Evaluation

In January 2003 I had my first visit with the psychologist, Hannah Merlock, at the Northeast Psychological Group in Concord. Her office was conveniently located near the hospital and my surgeon's office. The waiting room had a large open sitting area and a small enclosed play area. Two adults sat in the open area and another played with a child in the enclosed area. The receptionist, nurses, and office assistants were behind what appeared to be a bullet-proof glass partition. Bullet-proof came to mind because of all the warnings and cautionary notes taped to it and the fact that the window to the receptionist area was closed and locked.

I stood in front of the window for nearly 10 minutes before I was acknowledged. I do not like being ignored, especially when I am standing directly in front of someone who is doing nothing but looking at me. The receptionist looked at me and then turned away. I rang the bell. I felt invisible and was getting angry. She opened the glass window and bellowed, "Why are you here?"

"I have an appointment with Dr. Merlock," I responded matter-of-factly. She instructed me to have a seat until my name was called.

I felt uneasy. The comfort that I generally feel in most doctors' offices was replaced by fear. I had to calm myself as I looked around the room. I feared an attack or unpleasant scene would happen at any moment. I wondered if everyone around me had

severe psychiatric problems and if they thought I was crazy. I hoped I would not have to wait long.

The minute my name was called, I jumped to my feet and raced to the door where the assistant waited. She escorted me down and around a hallway to Dr. Merlock's office. The small office contained a desk and two chairs. A still life hung on the wall. Nothing in the room suggested anything about the doctor's personality or values.

Our conversation focused on my reasons for considering gastric bypass surgery. She asked questions about my relationships with my mother, father, and siblings, my job, my education, and what I understood about the weight-loss process. After speaking with her for approximately 20 minutes I was led into another small room that contained a table against the wall with a computer on top and a chair in front. There was another chair to the side of the table facing forward. I was instructed to sit at the computer and follow the instructions until the program informed me that I was finished.

On the computer was the Millon Behavioral Medicine Diagnostic test. This test is designed to measure one's level of stress, what types of coping strategies one is likely to use, how one responds to illness and pain, and how one is likely to utilize health care. I answered approximately 150 true/false questions. Many of the questions had nothing to do with decision-making around surgery. They focused on behaviors, primarily illegal behaviors such as drug use, and cognitions such as religious beliefs and trust. Some questions addressed one's interactions with other people. I felt the test fundamentally assessed whether one had evil thoughts and could possibly hurt oneself. I found the whole thing amusing more than anything else.

When I finished, an assistant took me back to the receptionist area. I was informed that I would be notified when my next visit would be scheduled after the psychologist reviewed the results of the test I had taken. My first visit with the psychologist was billed

as a diagnostic evaluation costing $175. Fortunately my co-payment was only $37.80.

The following month I had my second and final visit with the psychologist. She simply asked if anything had changed since the last time I saw her, which it had not, and indicated that the first test did not identify anything unusual. I was taken to the small room with the computer again. This time I had to answer approximately 350 of the same type of true/false questions. The Minnesota Multiphasic Personality Inventory-2 (MMPI-2) measures one's emotional, affective functioning, and coping behavior. This session was billed as an individual 45 to 50 minute therapy session at a cost of $150. I paid $39.20 out of pocket. I guess the second test did not identify anything unusual either, because I didn't hear from this office again.

During January 2003, Nell Carter, one of my favorite Broadway and television actresses, died at the age of 54. Nell Carter, who was African American, had been an overweight diabetic and had a brain aneurysm. I recalled her public service announcements about managing your diabetes and testing your blood sugar regularly. I remembered the media and tabloid reports of her battle with obesity. The news saddened me. My desire to lose weight increased.

First Visit with the Endocrinologist

Early in February 2003, I received a welcome letter, registration materials, and a pamphlet from The Endocrinology Clinic at Northeast Medical Center (NEMC), in preparation of my scheduled appointment with Dr. Abram Strauss. I was asked to arrive 15 minutes early to complete more registration paperwork. Copies of all my medical records and recent lab results were requested and required to be submitted at least one day before my appointment. It was suggested that I sign release forms with all of my doctors to

avoid delays and to bring all of my current medications, the completed registration forms, my co-payment, and my insurance card with me to my first appointment.

I liked the pamphlet. It explained the term "endocrinology." Endocrinology is the diagnosis and treatment of conditions affecting the body's endocrine system including the pituitary, thyroid, and adrenal glands. The pamphlet also noted that the doctors in the clinic were experts in the evaluation and management of diabetes, thyroid disease, and osteoporosis. Separate inserts with a picture of each doctor and his or her educational history were included. I was impressed that the clinic had both a woman and an African American man affiliated with it.

My endocrinologist, Dr. Abram Strauss, appeared to be 40-ish with beautiful curly hair and a reassuring smile. He had attended medical school at the State University of New York (SUNY) Health Science Center in Brooklyn, New York, and had completed his residency in internal medicine at the Albert Einstein College of Medicine at the Bronx Municipal Hospital Center. I knew he had to have had experience with African Americans, which was important to me.

An insert entitled "The Weight Management Program" addressed eating plans, lifestyle counseling, exercise, medical supervision, medical treatments, time commitments, and insurance issues. The following line impressed me the most: "Losing 10% or more is achievable, but losing down to your 'ideal' weight and keeping it off is not a realistic goal for most overweight people because of the genes associated with obesity. What counts is not how much you lose, but how much you keep off." This intuitively made sense to me and further validated my reasoning for having gastric bypass surgery. With the surgery I had a better chance of losing the maximum amount of weight possible and keeping a large portion of it off for the rest of my life. The surgery would provide me the opportunity to make an effective and healthy lifestyle change.

My first visit with my endocrinologist was the most intense of all my doctor visits. Dr. Strauss spoke fast and covered numerous issues. His instructions seemed to be based on the unspoken

assumption that I was a good candidate for gastric bypass surgery. He seemed especially concerned about my diabetes and hypertension and how they might impact my recovery immediately after surgery. To control my diabetes and hypertension, I already took three oral medications, but thankfully I didn't need to control my diabetes with insulin. Nevertheless, Dr. Strauss introduced me to insulin and had a nurse teach me how to use it in case of an emergency post-surgery. The nurse taught me how to give insulin using a round plastic object resembling an orange. The most important part of the lecture seemed to be getting the measurements right and getting the air out of the needle. I had to do it correctly twice before she felt that I knew what I was doing. I did not feel confident, and was afraid that I would forget this information rather quickly, but I kept my insecurity to myself. Then I realized I could get my sister, a nurse, to teach me the procedures again later. Plus, if anything happened to me after surgery and my sister was there— I would not have to do anything, she would definitely take control. Of this I was sure! Dr. Strauss gave me a packet with the instructions and tools to practice injecting insulin and a prescription for Humalog. He explained that he was giving me everything I needed then so I would be prepared post-surgery and would not have to call his office or come in for a prescription. It was "just in case."

In addition, Dr. Strauss insisted that I have an eye exam, since I had not had one in over a year, to help determine if the diabetes had already begun to damage my body in any way. He ordered an EKG and blood tests to evaluate my blood glucose levels and an ultrasound of my thyroid to look at a nodule he found while examining my throat and neck area. He spent 20 to 30 minutes feeling the right lower side of my neck. As he touched the area I could feel the shape of the nodule protruding out slightly. I nearly choked. He said it felt like "a small nut." My mind started racing. What the hell does he mean by "a small nut?" Are we talking peanut, walnut, or macadamia nut? I was too afraid to ask. I was not sure that I really wanted to know, at least not at that moment. I would try to determine this for myself later. "It is probably

nothing but I think we should have you checked for possible thyroid cancer," he said.

Cancer!? What a scary word! My mind raced again. Hell no! I do *not* have cancer! I know I *don't* have cancer! I knew it could *not* be true and I would have any tests my doctors felt necessary to prove it was not so.

"How often do you see cases of thyroid cancer?" I asked.

"Only three to four times a year," he responded nonchalantly.

That did not sound too bad. My mind raced—unless he only saw 3 to 4 individuals a year! Okay, don't be stupid, of course he sees hundreds of patients a year! Stop it! There is nothing to get excited about—yet!

Before leaving his office, I was given a pneumococcal vaccine that Dr. Strauss claimed "would prevent infection and pneumonia after surgery." On the way out of the clinic, I stopped by the receptionist window to have more lab tests scheduled and to pay my bill. The lab tests were scheduled for that very day! I was already late for my appointment with the nutritionist. The receptionist was kind enough to call her and let her know that I was running late and would be there within 10 minutes. This office visit cost $327.70. My co-payment was $77.54. Thank God for health insurance!

First Visit with the Nutritionist

Immediately after I left my endocrinologist's office I went to my scheduled appointment with the nutritionist, Dee Short, a registered nurse and certified lifestyle counselor with the Weight Management Program in Concord. The visit was short because my visit with the endocrinologist had run into our meeting time. Dee's assistant Amy greeted me when I arrived and escorted me to Dee's office. Amy requested the $100 payment due at the first visit and I gave her a check. The one-year program would cost me $500 out of pocket because it was not covered by my insurance company though required by my bariatric surgeon.

Dee introduced herself and showed me her wall covered with the before-and-after photos of women who had had weight-loss surgery. She briefly discussed the diet for gastric bypass patients post-surgery and presented me with lots of reading material and health assessment instruments to complete at home and mail in later. She said I would not need to see her again until after my surgery, but I should call the office as soon as I learned my surgery date. We didn't spend enough time with each other for me to get an idea of how well our relationship would work out.

After my visit with the nutritionist, I went to the Medical Arts Building to have the blood tests and thyroid ultrasound ordered by my endocrinologist. Then I went to the Cancer Center to have an EKG. Everything went smoothly, but it was a long day.

When I returned home, I found an intriguing letter in my mailbox. Apparently my bariatric surgeon and family doctor had a discussion about whether I should use the weight management program he, the bariatric surgeon endorsed, or the one she, my family doctor in Charlotte endorsed. Considering how expensive my office visits had been with her, I was convinced her program would have been much more expensive than the one I had already agreed to attend. I figured if I went with the program he endorsed, there would be more eyes on me that understood weight-loss surgery and the necessary aftercare required. His letter to her, which was copied to me, stated, "Thank you for offering to do the post-op nutrition management for Ms. Drummond. We do however have a formal one-year surgical weight program that all of the patients enroll in. We also have a diabetes protocol for patients such as Ms. Drummond. She will be enrolled in the program as per our usual routine."

Second Visit with Endocrinologist

In April 2003 I saw my endocrinologist, Dr. Abram Strauss, to do an aspiration of the nodule on my thyroid. A nurse presented me with

a consent form that I read and signed. Then she prepared me for the aspiration by numbing the area around the nodule. Once the area was numb, the doctor took a series of four needles and extracted cells from the nodule. Each needle was larger than the last. I am not needle-phobic, but the last needle did make the hair on my head rise and for some reason excited the muscles beneath my eyebrows. Dr. Strauss commented that the slides might have too much blood on them for proper analysis, which meant we might have to do another aspiration later, but he would send what he had to the laboratory and see what they said. He told me to call the office in a week for the results. I was in and out of the office in 30 minutes.

I was not afraid to hear the results but was a little apprehensive about what those results might actually reveal. With the diabetes and hypertension, I just did not want another health problem to address. To relieve my anxiety, I called Mac, my mother's best friend, a woman I think of as my second mom. Mac insisted that I did not have thyroid cancer and repeated over and over again, "You know how your body is! You have had cystic breasts and fibroids! That is just the nature of your body." I knew she was right. Mac is a religious woman; her faith is unshakable and undeniable. She prayed for me and had the answer. She prayed for me when I could not pray for myself. I did not have thyroid cancer. Yes, I knew she was right—this would not be an issue, and it wasn't an issue. A week later my endocrinologist's nurse practitioner told me that the nodule was benign. It would be left alone and "re-evaluated later."

DISCUSSION QUESTIONS

1. How should you prepare for a visit to the doctor's office? Nonverbally, what does the setup and aesthetics of an office tell you about the doctor and his or her practice and personality?

2. What do you think and feel when you see an overweight person? Why? What does this say about you as a person?

3. What role has specialization played in the health care of Americans, managed care, and health insurance?

4. How long does it take you to see your doctor once you have arrived for your appointment? Is there any evidence that the amount of time a doctor spends with you is directly or indirectly related to your health outcomes and satisfaction?

5. Are there differences between men and women and how they view excess weight?

6. Have you ever viewed a health video in your doctor's office or some other health facility? What did you like and dislike about the video? Explain.

7. What experiences have you had in a waiting room that disturbed you? Have you ever felt like your privacy rights were being violated? Explain. What did you do about it? What should you have done?

8. What role, if any, should psychological testing play in one's decision to have a particular surgical procedure?

9. Are you influenced by celebrities when making decisions about your health care? How? Why?

10. Is there any such thing as information overload? How much and what do we actually remember from our conversations with health professionals? How does medical jargon impact our understanding of a diagnosis and decision-making?

SUGGESTED READINGS

Doctor-Patient Communication

Cegala, D. L., Gade, C., Broz, S. L., & McClure, L. (2004). Physicians' and patients' perceptions of patients' communication competence in a primary care medical interview. *Health Communication, 16*(3), 289–305.

Gordon, H. S., Street Jr., R. L., Kelly, P. A., Souchek, J., & Wray, N. P. (2005). Physician-patient communication following invasive procedures: An analysis of post-angiogram consultations. *Social Science & Medicine, 61*(5), 1015–1025.

Santoso, J. T., Engle, D. B., Schaffer, L., & Wan, J. (2006). Cancer diagnosis and treatment: Communication accuracy between patients and their physicians. *Cancer Journal, 12*(1), 73–76.

Swenson, S. L., Buell, S., Zettler, P., White, M., Ruston, D. C., & Lo, B. (2004). Patient-centered communication: Do patients really prefer it? *Journal of General Internal Medicine, 19,* 1069–1079.

The Validity of Psychological Tests

Rustad, L. C. (1985). Testing the test. *Journal of Counseling and Development, 64*(4), 280–283.

A Team Approach to Health Care

Stille, C. J., Jerant, A., Bell, D., Meltzer, D., & Elmore, J. G. (2005). Coordinating care across diseases, settings, and clinicians: A key role for the generalist in practice. *Annals of Internal Medicine, 142*(8), 700–710.

Religion

Loren, M., Nesteruk, O., Swanson, M., Garrison, B., & Davis, T. (2005). Religion and health among African Americans. *Research on Aging, 27*(4), 447–474.

3

Laparoscopic Gastric Bypass Surgery

Surgery Is Scheduled

Robin, the surgery scheduler, called at the end of March 2003 to place me on the calendar for surgery. She wanted to give me a date in April, but I told her school would still be in session which meant I would not be able to take three or more weeks off. I suggested a date in May. She gave me a tentative date of May 12, and she suggested I call back in the middle of April for verification.

On April 28 I called the office. Robin was no longer employed with the clinic, so my call was directed to the new surgery scheduler. She told me that my surgery was scheduled for noon on May 27, 2003. Before the surgery I would have to have a presurgery meeting with the surgeon and another with hospital admission personnel. We discussed possible dates and times and settled on Wednesday, May 21. My hospital admission date was confirmed in a letter from my health insurance company.

Presurgery Interview with Surgeon

My second meeting with my bariatric surgeon was more relaxed than our first encounter. We were both obviously excited to move

forward with the surgery. Dr. Bozeman summarized the findings of the preoperative tests I had taken. The tests confirmed I was experiencing some of the key co-morbidities of obesity, including diabetes, hypertension, gastric reflux disease, and high cholesterol. Additionally, the psychological tests indicated I had good coping abilities, while the endocrinologist's report suggested I would benefit greatly from such surgery. "We are ready to proceed," Dr. Bozeman said. "If you don't have any questions about the procedure and want to have the surgery, then I need you to read the consent form very carefully and sign it. Take as much time as you need."

During my first visit at the clinic, I was given a copy of the consent form and had read and reread it several times over the past three to four months. There is truth in the statement that we see something different each and every time we read something. Even though I was intimately familiar with the document, it felt as if I was reading it for the first time. Its significance did not escape me. The seven-page single-spaced consent form was entitled "Special Informed Consent for the Laparoscopic (Roux-En-Y) Gastric Bypass." At the top were spaces for the patient's name and age. The first paragraph indicated that it was a legal document and instructed the patient to initial next to each paragraph and the bottom right corner of each page to signify explicitly that the information had been read and understood.

A consent form is intended to be written verification of the discussions a patient has with her surgeon about the procedure and its benefits and risks. This document did just that. It explained the procedure and its possible benefits, especially its ability to eliminate or improve various co-morbidities. One section specified the number of procedures preformed by the specialist of the clinic and the complication rate. Then the following risks were enumerated and described: allergic reactions, anesthetic complications, bleeding, blood clots, infection, leaks, narrowing/stricture, indigestion, dumping syndrome, bowel obstruction, laparoscopic surgery risks,

side effects of drugs, loss of bodily function, risks of transfusion, hernia, hair loss, vitamin and mineral deficiencies, inadequate weight loss, excessive weight loss, unplanned pregnancy, complications of pregnancy, depression, and death. There was even a section to address the possibility that other complications might arise that were previously unrecognized.

The decision to have gastric bypass surgery should not be taken lightly. Death is a possibility just as it is a possibility with any type of minor or major surgery. As the consent form noted, "This is a major and serious operation. It may lead to death from complications in some circumstances. There has been a death in the first week after this type of surgery in one patient." I assumed this statement referred to one of my doctor's patients, but did not verify.

In my mind, the risks of hair loss and malnutrition were just as threatening. After watching my mother age 30 years during the two years she fought and lost the battle to complications of diabetes and hypertension, I knew what malnutrition looked like. She did not want to eat and at times could not eat. Her body betrayed her. She went from walking and standing under her own strength to using a cane, a wheelchair, and, in the end, being bedridden. I had witnessed her thick, jet-black, easily managed hair become thin, gray, coarse, and unmanageable. Imagine how I felt knowing that I was purposely choosing to restrict the absorption of nutrients in my body by having my stomach and intestine manipulated. My hair had always been the source of my vanity, and it was already thinning. Did I really want to intensify my rate of hair loss in a matter of months? My decision to have weight-loss surgery was not made lightly. I truly understood the risks.

The last few pages of the consent form addressed the need to commit to long-term care and follow-up visits with the surgeon for years, and the danger of leaving the immediate area too soon after surgery. There was an acknowledgement that I had been informed about similar weight-loss procedures and an authorization for the release of my medical information to educate other

patients. I signed the document. It was witnessed by a nurse and signed by Dr. Bozeman. As I prepared to leave the office, I was given a packet called the "Patient Manual for Gastric Bypass" and instructed to familiarize myself with its contents immediately. Smiling, Dr. Bozeman and I looked into each other's eyes for several seconds as we shook hands and said our silent good-byes. I paid my $15 co-payment and left the office ready and hopeful.

Preoperative Interview at Hospital

When I left Dr. Bozeman's office, I crossed the street to the Surgery Center at NEMC. The receptionist at the information desk directed me to the admissions office. There, I was advised, a nurse would discuss North Carolina law concerning advance directives and the purpose of ethics committees and an anesthesiologist would need to verify specific information about me. The nurse did not have much to say about advance directives or the purpose of ethics committees. She simply instructed me to go to Pastoral Care if I wanted information on living wills and handed me a pamphlet entitled "Advance Directives and Ethics Committees." Fortunately, I was already familiar with the concept of living wills and ethics committees. I recalled vividly the moment my mother signed her living will as we sat in her attorney's office just 4 months before her death. That experience lead to many discussions between me and my siblings about what we desired to happen for ourselves. I did not want any unusual means taken to prolong my life. I did not want to exist in a vegetative state, receive resuscitation, or be placed on dialysis if my kidneys failed. My sister would see to my wishes, if and when necessary, as she saw to our mother's.

The nurse did a much better job explaining the preoperative patient instructions. She asked, "How do you learn best—through pictures or through reading?"

As an educator I knew both means were good ways to learn. Both had advantages and disadvantages. I thought about it for a few seconds. "I like both, but if I had to choose only one, it would be reading."

She handed me a form with my preoperative instructions and gave me an opportunity to read it. When I finished reading, she reiterated its contents, "You must cease the use of all medications the day before surgery except for the Diovan, the anti-hypertension drug, which you will have to take the morning of surgery. Stop eating by midnight before the surgery and understand that if you don't follow these instructions, the surgery could be postponed or cancelled. You must also have a responsible adult to drive you home upon discharge."

She concluded by quickly summarizing the general instructions that apply to all admitted patients including what to wear, what to do if I got a cold, to leave all valuables at home, and to wear no makeup, contact lenses, or hair accessories on the day of surgery. I signed the form and she gave me a copy. The form indicated my surgery had been moved up from noon to 7:30 a.m. with a check-in time of 5:45 a.m. A good omen—this pleased me greatly because I am a morning person.

The week leading up to my surgery was quiet. I packed my bags, cleaned the house, read and reread all of the literature I had on the procedure, and dreamed about the day when I could claim freedom from diabetes and hypertension. The majority of my time was spent shopping with one of my best friends, Rana, who arrived in town from Kentucky. My sister, Marlene, came from Conover, North Carolina, the evening before my surgery after working a hospital shift, and together we prepared for the big day. Even though my actions and conversations with Rana and Marlene in previous weeks may have suggested that I did not need anyone, their company and support were greatly appreciated. I did not want to be alone.

Countdown: 24 Hours and Waiting

The day before surgery I mixed Fleets Phospho Soda, a laxative, with 4 ounces of water and drank it. I followed that with 8 ounces of water. What nasty stuff! From that point on, I did not drink or eat anything else. To decrease the risk of bleeding during surgery, I did not take any aspirin or aspirin-containing medicines, even though my mouth and gums were irritated. One tablet of the antibiotic Levoquin and two tablets of Prevacid were taken at 10:00 p.m. with just a sip of water. Before going to bed, I washed my body with a red liquid antiseptic called Hibiclens and placed one anti-nausea Transderm Scop patch on the hairless area behind my left ear. I tried unsuccessfully to sleep.

At approximately 4:30 a.m. I took one Reglan pill to treat gastric reflux and my anti-hypertension drug, Diovan, as instructed by the anesthesiologist. I washed my body once again with the Hibiclens and dressed comfortably in jeans and a t-shirt. It was Tuesday, May 27, 2003, the day of my surgery. As Marlene drove Rana and I the 20 minutes to Concord, I thought about the 6½ months since I first met with my surgeon and begun this journey. I was happy, anxious, excited, and strangely at peace.

The Hospital Stay

When we arrived at the check-in section of the Surgery Center at NEMC, no one was there to greet us. We sat down and waited. Others arrived and joined us in the waiting area. The receptionist arrived around 6:00 a.m. and asked for the first arrival to join her. I sat directly across from her. She smiled and joked about how much difficulty she had getting up that morning. I gave her my name, which she located on a sheet in front of her, then requested my surgery account payment. I handed her a check made payable to the hospital for $20. Her request was not a surprise. I had

received a phone call nearly a week before informing me that I would be required to make a payment to the hospital on the day of admittance. It was explained to me that I, and not my insurance company, would be solely responsible for the payment of my surgery account of approximately $1,300. In that phone conversation I agreed to make a payment of $20.00 on the day of surgery and to make monthly payments of $150 until the account was paid off.

Next the receptionist gave me a copy of NEMC's Notice of Privacy Practices and asked, "Who would you like to stay with you as you prepare for surgery?"

"My sister and friend are here with me," I answered.

"You can only have one visitor with you at a time, so decide who will go first and then the other will be able to join you later." Marlene and Rana decided that Marlene would go back with me first. The receptionist instructed an aide to take us to the prep area.

In the prep area I removed all of my clothes and jewelry except for the earring in the tragus of my left ear and put on a hospital gown and cap. I laid on the gurney, and my sister covered me with blankets. The earring in the tragus of my left ear was purchased nearly five years earlier after I had completed graduate school and returned to North Carolina. Marlene had gotten one done first, and after getting her reassurance that it was not as painful as it looked, I went with her to a tattoo parlor to have it done. For me the earring symbolized both the bond between us and the completion of a major goal in my life—graduate school. The design of the earring required pliers for its removal and I thought no one would object to one small earring remaining in my ear. Nevertheless, three nurses looked at my ear and insisted that the earring be removed. One finally figured out a way to pull the earring apart and handed it to my sister. Marlene took possession of all of my belongings and placed them in a plastic bag.

For several minutes we remained in the curtained-off area alone until joined by Rana. We noticed one of my nurses had my first name and the other my middle name spelled the exact same

way, and we saw this as a good omen. As a precaution, one of the nurses, Darlene, asked me directly what my name was and what type of surgery I was there for. Then a member of the anesthesiology team came in and tried to put an IV in my left hand. He tried numerous times and failed. Red-faced with embarrassment, he admitted he could not seem to get the IV into my left hand and had to try the right hand. He was successful but neglected to stop the bleeding where he punctured me on the left hand. My sister got some gauze from one of the nurses and took care of it once he left.

I am not afraid of needles and his awkwardness did not bother me. Rana, however, was disturbed by his inability to get it right the first time. She nervously paced the floor and repeated over and over again, "Needles don't bother you, huh."

At approximately 7:25 a.m., I was wheeled into the operating room. I must have gone under on the way, because I do not remember the room or who was present.

Nearly 3 hours later, in my private room on the second floor of the hospital, I awakened as a nurse removed the catheter used to collect urine from my urethra. Marlene and Rana waited outside the door until the nurse told them to come in. After greetings, hugs, and kisses, they sat with me. Marlene had spoken with my surgeon, Dr. Bozeman, who said the surgery had gone smoothly even though the scar tissue from my decade-old hysterectomy challenged him. I was extremely tired and do not remember much of my conversation with them. I was not allowed to eat or drink anything. I slept much of the afternoon and evening away.

Marlene and Rana were determined I would get up and walk, as instructed by my doctor, before the day ended. They helped me into two hospital gowns to cover my front and backside sufficiently, wrapped the cords around my monitor, and escorted me around the floor, lap after lap. When we returned to the room, they placed the compression stockings, which are designed to decrease the risk of blood clotting, back on my legs and replugged all of the cords back into the wall that were connected to my mon-

itor. Sometime that evening a staff doctor came into the room and told me that the operation had gone well. I slept.

On the second day I began a liquid diet with chocolate-flavored Glycerna. I was instructed to drink as much as I could to get in the 45 grams of protein I needed. To do that I would have to drink 4½ cans with 12 ounces each for a total of 54 ounces of protein drink. Plus, I was required to follow each serving of protein with water. I was told to drink 30 cc's of water for every 60 cc's of protein drink. Each day I tried to drink as much as I could but never achieved the minimum of 45 grams of protein during my hospital stay. It took me all day to make it through two cans. Thankfully, my release was not based on my ability to drink the required amount of liquids. The hospital staff didn't *know* about my failure to drink the required amounts of liquid, because they never checked nor documented my intake. My nutritionist, Dee, did come by, reiterated the importance of protein, congratulated me for what I was able to drink and encouraged me to drink more. We arranged to meet on June 10 to discuss further the nutritional plan I would have to follow.

For the next 3 days, my blood sugar and blood pressure were taken at least four times a day. My blood sugar went from a high of 187 immediately after surgery to 94 on the day of my release. Dr. Hoffman from the surgical unit informed me my diabetes was apparently cured and I would not need to take any diabetes-related medications anymore. In addition, my blood pressure remained below 130/70 and I would not have to take the anti-hypertension drug, Diovan. Yes, my primary goal to never have to take prescription medications again had been achieved!

I expected to be released from the hospital the day after my surgery, but my temperature was erratic, ranging from 97.7 to 101.7. As a precaution, my surgeon insisted I stay another day. I was disappointed but respected my doctor for looking out for my best interests. Rana commented that my disappointment was clearly evident on my face.

Even though I loved having my sister and best friend spend the first two nights with me, I began to realize that I wasn't getting much sleep. Part of the reason was that everyone kept readjusting the temperature in the room. Rana is cold-natured and wanted the temperature to be at least 80 degrees. I am hot-natured and wanted the room temperature to be between 70 and 75 degrees. On my last night in the hospital, alone and with the room temperature approximately 70 degrees, I slept well! My sister returned home to work and Rana spent the night in my apartment. I encouraged Rana to go out and have fun, and she did. Shawn, a colleague and friend of ours, took her on a tour of downtown Charlotte and out to dinner. They brought me "get well" balloons and cards when they returned to visit the next day.

On the third day of my stay in the hospital, I had X-rays of my chest and abdomen area and another upper GI series. I thought I was going to die if I had to swallow another drop of barium. I did observe that they were careful to mix much less than I had during my GI series before surgery; the technician did not pressure me to drink a lot. The first time I had this series I was prone on the machine, and this time I stood the entire time. I think this had something to do with my incisions and drain getting in the way of imaging, and trying to decrease the amount of strain on my body with constant position changes. This test determined that I was ready for release from the hospital. It confirmed the surgery had gone well and I did not have any punctures or leaks in my abdomen.

Overall, my hospital stay was routine. Most of the time I was alone or in the company of Rana. The nurses during the day shift were attentive to me, my family, and friends, but after 7:00 p.m. I rarely saw any of the nursing staff. During the night shift, I did not see anyone until around 5:45 a.m., when my blood pressure was taken, blood sugar level assessed, and I was given Prevacid, Levoquin, and Carafate, all in the span of 2 minutes. One care-partner (CP) assisted me in washing my back twice during my stay, but otherwise I was on my own. Only once did a nurse change the

dressing around my incisions. That was on the first day. Unfortunately, she did not work the remainder of my stay. All the other nurses simply looked at the Jackson-Pratt drain to see how full it was and occasionally emptied it. I was responsible for getting my walks in, washing up, getting to the bathroom safely, getting nutrition, cleaning up my room, packing my bags, and making my discharge arrangements. It was extremely helpful to have family and friends with me. They were my true caregivers.

One alarming event did occur during my stay. A white elderly male patient burst into my room as I was in the process of washing up. He stared at my nakedness and yelled, "I thought this was my room!"

I responded with anger, "It clearly is not, so please leave!"

He stood there frozen and staring. I covered my body with a towel, walked toward him as he blocked the entrance to the room, and screamed, "Get the hell out of my room!"

He left. Even though we were yelling and screaming at the tops of our lungs, no hospital staff came to investigate what was happening. Later that day I told the CP about the incident. She apologized and confided that the man had serious mental problems. Apparently he was causing all kinds of problems for the nursing staff and they spent a great deal of time chasing him around the floor. That night he was moved to another floor.

DISCUSSION QUESTIONS

1. What does it mean to consent to surgery? What is the purpose of a consent form? What should a consent form include? What rights do patients have in changing or amending a consent form?

2. How do we view hair in our culture? How do we talk about hair texture, thinning or loss? Are there cultural differences in how hair is valued and discussed? What significance does hair,

or the lack thereof, play in the maintenance or transformation of one's self-concept?

3. Have you planned for your death? Why or why not? How should you discuss your death with loved ones? What is an advance directive? When should one get one and what should it contain? What, if any, legal differences exist between states in the content requirements of such documents?

4. What is an ethics committee? What role does an ethics committee play in your decision to have surgery? How are your rights, values, beliefs, and concerns advocated and addressed by an ethics committee? What are some differences between states' requirements and standards for these committees?

5. How do you learn best? Are there cultural differences in the way we learn?

6. How does socioeconomic status impact health care?

7. What privacy rights do patients have while in the hospital? How should problems with other patients be handled?

SUGGESTED READINGS

Consent Issues

Dixon-Woods, M., Williams, S. J., Jackson, C. J., Akkad, A., Kenyon, S., & Habiba, M. (2006). Why do women consent to surgery, even when they do not want to? An interactionist and Bourdieusian analysis. *Social Science & Medicine, 62*(11), 2742–2753.

Epstein, M. (2006). Why effective consent presupposes autonomous authorization: A counterorthodox argument. *Journal of Medical Ethics, 32*(6), 342–345.

Socio-Economic Concerns

Ray, G. B. (2005). Medical care, health insurance, and family resources: Complications to otherwise good news. In E. B. Ray (Ed.), *Health communication in practice: A case study approach* (pp. 261–270). Mahwah, NJ: Lawrence Erlbaum Associates.

African American Hair and Body Image

Duke, L. (2000). Black in a blonde world: Race and girl's interpretations of the feminine ideal in teen magazines. *Journalism and Mass Communication Quarterly, 77*(2), 367–392.

Patton, T. O. (2006). Hey girl, am I more than my hair?: African American women and their struggles with beauty, body image, and hair. *NWSA Journal, 18*(2), 24–51.

Learning Styles

Jocson, K. M. (2006). "Bob Dylan and hip hop": Intersecting literacy practices in youth poetry communities. *Written Communication, 23*(3), 231–259.

Postma, L. (2001). A theoretical argumentation and evaluation of South African learners' orientation towards and perceptions of the empowering use of information: A calculated prediction of computerized learning for the marginalized. *New Media & Society, 3*(3), 313–326.

Rehling, L. (2005). Teaching in a high-tech conference room: Academic adaptations and workplace simulations. *Journal of Business and Technical Communication, 19*(1), 98–113.

4

Week One Post-Surgery

First Day Home

FRIDAY, MAY 30, 2003. While still in the hospital, I was concerned whether or not I had enough money in my bank account to cover all of the checks I wrote in the days preceding the operation to cover prescriptions and the purchase of protein drinks, ice pops, sugar-free Jell-O, and Crystal Light that I needed for 2 weeks postoperatively. As I thought about how to juggle funds around, the phone rang. It was Rana. She had spent the night at my apartment and was calling to find out how I planned to get home.

My understanding was that Rana would come by the hospital with Shawn to see me home after being discharged. Shawn would drive because Rana could not drive my car, which is a stick shift. All she mentioned was taking a run and a shower and preparing for her return to Kentucky. Shawn would take her to the airport later that evening. She asked what I did that morning, and I told her I walked, bathed, dressed, and had the IV removed.

Then she asked, "Do you have someone to pick you up? I will probably be here when you get here, but I need to go to the drugstore and pick up my medication, the Z-Pak."

My heart raced. "No!" I mouthed softly to myself but responded out loud, "Oh, sure, I have co-workers who live in Concord who are probably headed toward the campus area. It won't be a problem for one of them to pick me up."

"Okay, I will see you later."

For the next hour and a half I stressed over calling the Lee-mans, my department chair and his wife. I called their home. No answer. Carol Leeman is active in her community, especially with her children's school activities, and probably would not be immediately available to me. I called the office. Our receptionist, Mary, answered and immediately began to patch me through to Dr. Richard Leeman. I hung up the phone. I just could not ask my boss for a favor.

Panicking, I called others that might help me out—Cheryl S., Cheryl E., Shawn—but they did not answer their phones and I did not leave any messages. Ten minutes later I called my boss again and told the secretary that we had been disconnected. Of course, she had tried immediately to reach me after the "disconnect" and was upset that it had happened.

"Do you have a cold?" she asked.

"No, just a little congestion."

Why didn't I ask her for help? I knew she or our administrative assistant, Pat, would come to my aide. But I just couldn't ask either. I did not want to appear weak to my co-workers. Therefore, I denied them the opportunity to assist me. Mary put me through to Dr. Leeman.

"Rich, this is Darlene Drummond and I have been hospitalized for the past 4 days at NEMC having had major surgery. Is it possible for you or Carol to pick me up when I'm discharged sometime in the next hour?" He responded that he had to meet with an adjunct faculty member and would not be able to but would contact his wife and leave a message with her. He wanted assurance that I was okay. I told him I was fine and gave him the phone number to my hospital room and waited.

During the wait I realized that I didn't even have enough cash with me to take a taxi home. I would need at least $40. I called other co-workers and acquaintances. None were available. More than 30 minutes passed before I heard from Carol. She reassured me that she would do everything in her power to help me.

I packed my bags, straightened up the room, and cleaned the bathroom. A nurse brought me the discharge papers. She looked over the four-page document and said, "All this stuff was probably discussed between you and your surgeon. You need to fill these prescriptions when you leave, and sign here that I have gone over this information with you." I read the four pages and signed my name. Once the nurse collected the paperwork, a small but strong elderly man pushed me in a wheelchair to the Surgery Center discharge and pickup area.

Carol met me there. This busy mother of two took her boys to their swimming lessons, assisted the PTA in setting up their end-of-the-school-year party, and then arrived at the hospital at 11:30 a.m. to pick me up. As we took Highway 29 through the university area to my residence, I told Carol why I was in the hospital and apologized for not telling her and other members of the faculty and staff sooner. She told me that she would be available to assist me with anything I needed, such as grocery shopping and rides to see members of my health-care team. She agreed to pick me up and take me back to Concord for an appointment with my surgeon on Tuesday, June 5, to have my drain removed.

When we arrived at the apartment complex, Carol graciously carried my bags up three flights of stairs. I climbed the stairs without any problems, and it felt good to know that my body was strong. Rana greeted us at the door and helped us get the bags inside. After Carol left, Rana went for her morning run to Eckerd Drugs to fill her prescription. She brought back some sugar-free popsicles and immediately began to clear out all the meat, frozen vegetables, ice-cream, and other foods from my refrigerator. Only bottled water, vanilla-flavored Ensure, chocolate-flavored Boost, vanilla-flavored Kashi Go-Lean, and a pitcher of Tropical Passions Crystal Light remained.

I was not ready to go to bed. I prepared the living room area by removing all of the pillows from the sofa and covering it with a sheet and blanket. I laid there and watched television for hours until Shawn arrived to pick up Rana to take her to the airport.

When they left, I watched my favorite afternoon program, *The Oprah Winfrey Show.*

You can't help but admire Oprah. Her show was in honor of the balladeer Luther Vandross and addressed preventing health disease and diabetes in the African American community. Luther had been in the hospital for nearly a month due to complications from his high blood pressure and diabetes. As his mother talked about the prevalence of diabetes in her family and Oprah enumerated the African American stars with diabetes, I couldn't help but think about my mother's battle with diabetes. My stifled cries turned into violent sobbing as I looked at her photograph on the television stand, hoping she knew I had learned something from her life and her death and that my surgery was evidence of this. I worked off my nervous energy by walking around the apartment and fixing up my bed for the night.

Before I settled in, I was able to drink enough protein shakes to get in 27 grams of protein, even though I had been told I needed a minimum of 45 grams a day. It took me until 10:00 p.m. to get that much down, and it began to dawn on me that I would have to find a better way to get the required grams per day. Happy to be back in my own bed, I quickly fell asleep. At approximately 3:00 a.m., I awoke with an irritated, sore, and dry mouth. I used the toilet, brushed my teeth and rinsed my mouth with the new Biotene products I had purchased before surgery, which helped. I went back to bed, only to get up once again to use the toilet.

The Rest of the First Week

MAY 31, 2003. I got up and immediately went to the bathroom to rinse my mouth. I was worried that my braced teeth may not survive this constant drama with dry mouth. Would my investment in braces backfire?

I touched my gown and realized that there was a big wet spot just below my right breast. My first thought was that it was blood

from the drain—maybe I had punctured that drainage "bulb suction" thing also known as the "Jackson Pratt." *Who in the hell is Jackson Pratt?* I thought about searching the Web to find out more about him. I did not know if I wanted to thank him or kill him.

As I sat on the toilet, I used toilet paper to squeeze the wet spot on my gown to determine what it was. It was yellow. *Did I urinate on myself and not realize it? I will be embarrassed if this happens while I am out in public.* I examined the drain, which was wet on the bottom but wasn't leaking. It was then that I realized that it had to be leakage from the incision site itself. This scared me because this had not happened while I was in the hospital. *Was I really aware about what was happening in this area? They had emptied my drain fewer than three times.* I grabbed the information manual given me at discharge that I kept on the sink in easy reach. The "Drain Care Instructions at Home Guide" stated, "Fluid leakage from the incision site is common. The fluid should be clear to pink to light yellow in color. If the fluid is bright red or becomes tan, thick, or has a foul odor, notify your doctor immediately." The leakage was yellow in color, so I tried to calm down.

The instructions stated that the site should be washed with soap and warm water once or twice a day and the dressing changed and replaced with clean, dry pieces of gauze on top of the site as often as needed. I took the easy way out and began piling on gauze with tape to keep it in place. Less than 2 hours later I looked at the site again and discovered more leakage. I panicked and called my sister, Marlene, who tried her best to reassure me that this was normal and nothing to be concerned about. She instructed me to remove all of the tape and gauze and wash the area. I couldn't do it. I piled on more gauze instead.

The more I piled on, the heavier the area seemed to be, and the more my concern about unpleasant body odor grew. I took, as one of my friends, Kai, phrases it, "a whore's bath" by standing at the sink and washing under my arms, breasts, between my legs, and around my rectum area. I felt fresher, but not as fresh as when I've had a shower. A shower—I really wanted and needed a

shower but I was not ready to attempt one with a drain hanging from my abdomen.

Most of the morning was spent focusing on drinking as many protein shakes as possible and drinking water to prevent dehydration. In between my periods of water and protein consumption, I would go to the bathroom mirror and peak at the incision area. I soon tired of this behavior and started to plan how I would get to the drugstore to get my prescriptions filled.

The doctors provided prescriptions for five medications that they thought I might need. Two prescriptions—Mepergan Fortis and Bextra—were for pain and were to be used only as needed. Obviously my doctors were interested in managing pain. In the hospital, however, I had not used much of the morphine prescribed immediately after surgery. In fact, the morphine was removed from my room the morning of the second day. Since I really had not experienced much pain throughout my hospital stay, I decided not to fill these prescriptions.

In addition, I was given a prescription for Phenergan and directed to use it via the rectum as needed for nausea. I knew that I wasn't going to fill that either. I just wasn't going to stick something up my rectum. Plus, I already had a prescription for Transderm Scop, which had successfully addressed my nausea problem in the past, and to use it I only had to place a small patch behind my ear every 3 days. This was definitely more pleasant than using a suppository.

The remaining two prescriptions would be filled. Both medications were introduced to me during my hospital stay. Carafate, a liquid, is used to protect the lining of the stomach. I would have to take 2 teaspoons three times a day. Levaquin, an antibiotic used to treat bacterial infections, would be taken once a day every day for 1 week only.

I called around to see who could take me to the drugstore, but no one was available. When my sister called, I was in tears bemoaning my lonely status in Charlotte. I believed everyone

expected a single, well-educated, African American woman to take care of herself. And that is exactly what I had done for years. Yet, today was different because I felt not only alone but lonely. I wanted someone to take care of me. Was this a legitimate way to feel even though I did not consider myself sick? I just wanted someone to acknowledge that they recognized I was not as strong as I pretended and that I really did not mind being dependent on others at times such as these.

My concerned sister called our "second mom" Mac, and told her that I was depressed. I was. I cried every time I piled on new clean gauze. Mac called one of her daughters, Jeanne, who lives in Charlotte less than 15 minutes from me. Jeanne and one of her nursing friends came to the house, picked me up, and took me to the credit union to get cash, and then took me to two different drugstores to fill my prescriptions. They did this in heavy rain during a tornado watch.

I told them about my surgery. Jeanne's immediate reaction was to note that the surgery is considered preventive in nature and paid for by the state's health plan. I appreciated this because I thought this indicated that they understood my decision to have the surgery. But then they started talking about another of their friends who had the surgery. She did not have any co-morbidities such as diabetes and hypertension but had been morbidly obese since childhood.

"She has lost a great deal of weight and looks so different now." This phrase was repeated over and over again, but I couldn't assess whether they believed this was good or bad. I know I didn't like it when they informed me that she claimed to eat anything she wanted and that they had seen her eat a large slice of strawberry shortcake soon after surgery. They commented that she was still losing weight—in their opinion, too much weight.

Is this a cultural phenomenon? When blacks look at one another, do they see the weight or size of the other differently than whites? How is it that when we think someone looks healthy, they

are usually overweight by current health standards? I, too, enjoy having a curvy body with a small waist, large thighs, hips, and buttocks. I am now, however, at the point where being healthy is much more important to me than having an hourglass figure, especially if that hourglass is running out of time!

We returned to my apartment and Jeanne offered to clean and dress my site. Rather than let her, I decided to challenge myself. It took 30 to 45 minutes as I removed slowly each piece of tape and gauze, but I did it and it wasn't as bad as I thought. I washed the area with soapy water, dried it, and dressed it with new gauze and tape. My pride in my accomplishment must have been evident to everyone who called to check in on me, including my sister, Mac, out-of-state friends, and Jeanne. All commented on how much better I sounded. Throughout the remainder of the day I practiced deep breathing exercises and purposely coughed to improve my lung capacity. And even though I got in only 28 grams of protein and not nearly enough water, I slept well.

SUNDAY, JUNE 01, 2003. A quiet day for me. I concentrated on reaching my 45 grams of protein per day goal and increasing the amount of clear liquids drunk, drinking less Crystal Light and more pure water. I noticed that the more liquid protein I consumed, the drier my mouth seemed. Nevertheless, I am sure that the consumption of more protein and water is the key to feeling better and maintaining energy. By the end of the day I had managed 40 grams of protein and 60 cc's of clear liquid.

That evening Rana called to checkup on me. She said her church was praying for me and she would pray for God to give me the right words as I wrote about my experience. I worried about her because she was going the next day to have yet another biopsy on a lump found in her breast. I wished I could be there for her.

MONDAY, JUNE 02, 2003. My sister called and I actually felt better when I realized what a great mood she was in. Marlene had spoken with one of the bariatric surgeons at the hospital where she

works about our family history and the possibility of having weight-loss surgery herself, getting her adolescent daughter ready for such surgery, and convincing her husband that this could change positively the quality of his life. I knew that my success in this endeavor could greatly impact the decision-making of others in my family. Since the death of our mother, our interest in leading a healthier lifestyle has increased.

After my conversation with Marlene, I got dressed and decided to take a walk outside. My goal was to go to the mail center of my complex and return to climb the three flights of stairs back to my apartment. I wore a big flannel shirt and loose pants with the drain secured to the flannel top. As I walked, I could feel the wind blow through my top, which made my incision area itch. I convinced myself that the air on the incision was a good thing. It would lead to faster healing and keep me smelling fresh. By the time I returned to the apartment my arms and upper shoulder areas hurt and felt heavy. A walk that would generally take me approximately 8 minutes took 13. Plus, it caused more leakage around the incision and I had to clean and redress it. This time I used less tape and gauze so the area would not feel as heavy.

I noticed that my vision was changing. I could see great at far distances with my glasses, but my vision at shorter distances didn't seem right. It was more difficult to read and write with my glasses on. *Is this normal?* I wondered, making a mental note to ask my doctor the next day.

Wow! Black people, especially if they are friends or acquaintances, hate it when you do not let them help you in your time of need. This realization hit home when I received a phone call from Cheryl E. I called Cheryl while in the hospital but was unable to give her the details of my situation because she was in the middle of a meeting and could not talk. I promised to call her back in 15 minutes, but didn't. After I apologized for not returning her call, I told her about my surgery. Cheryl lives less than 10 minutes from me and was upset that I hadn't allowed her to assist me.

"You know, I want a sister here in Charlotte. I consider *you* my sister here in Charlotte, and you didn't call me!?" I could hear the disappointment in her voice and felt bad, really bad, about not confiding in her.

"Are you alone?" she asked.

"Yes," I replied.

"I could come through this phone! I could come through this phone!" What is your address?" she demanded. I gave her my address and apologized over and over again for not telling her sooner, and she promised to be by to see me that afternoon. Cheryl and I had developed a professional relationship for nearly 3 years. We are both interested in and working toward improving the lives, overall well-being, and health of the African-American community. For months she had gone out of her way to include me in her life, but I had been my usual standoffish self! Oh God, why do I insist on doing things alone! Why do I make it difficult to be my friend? Why can I not accept that there are people out there who care about me?

Within 10 minutes of speaking with Cheryl, I received a call from Jeanne. She called to tell me that one of her co-workers who had the surgery also had the same surgeon! Ms. Jones wanted me to call her as soon as possible to talk about the first 2 to 3 weeks post-surgery. She believed I would be depressed and would want to speak with someone who had been through the surgery and dealt with depression. Jeanne gave me Ms. Jones's work, home, and cell phone numbers and told me to call at any time. Exactly what I needed—another African American woman who had the surgery to talk to! Thank you, Jeanne!

Late that afternoon, Cheryl came by. I got dressed and she drove me to the nearest drugstore to get more gauze, sugar-free Jell-O, and a different flavor of protein drink. Vanilla is nasty! But all of the other flavors, banana, Dutch chocolate, and French vanilla, contained only 9 to 11 grams of protein per serving. I ended up purchasing butter pecan with 13 grams of protein per serving. I knew I would eventually have to buy protein powder

from a major health food store and mix my own combinations to get many more grams of protein per serving.

We returned to my place, and talked about our dream and plan to come up with an intervention program to address health disparities and chronic illnesses such as obesity, diabetes, and cardiovascular disease in the African American community. When Cheryl left, I spent the rest of the evening deep breathing, coughing, watching television, and looking forward to having the drain removed the next day. The one thing that really bothered me was the aftertaste left in my mouth each time I drank a protein shake. My mouth was dry and I could swear I feel bacteria growing. I knew if I drank more water, my mouth would feel fresher, but how could I do that *and* get in the amount of protein grams I need? It wasn't easy!

That day I consumed only 25 grams of protein. I had to drink 360 cc's, or 12 ounces, of protein drink to get this amount which is no way near what my nutritionist instructed me to get. I was only able to get in 95 cc's of water, which was approximately 7 ounces. I had a lot of work to do to improve my nutritional intake. I hadn't felt hungry nor did I think about solid foods, but when I heard the gas rumbling in my stomach or I felt something in my throat, I felt the need to slow down on my intake. Nevertheless, in trying to fulfill the necessary nutritional requirements, I am drinking nearly every second of the day.

The day and week ended with checkup calls from Marlene and Mac. Mac laughingly reassured me, "If you need anything, anything at all, please call Jeanne." I could hear the smile behind this statement. My mother and Mac, not biological sisters, were true sisters in every sense of the word. Her children were my mothers and vice versa. As their children, we grew up together and as adults still kept in touch, although not as much as we should. I felt protected and loved, so loved that I called Rana to see how her breast biopsy turned out. No answer. Worried, I called Carol and reminded her to pick me up at 10:30 a.m. for my doctor's appointment.

DISCUSSION QUESTIONS

1. What types of support do you give family, friends, and co-workers when they are going through a health crisis? Are there any differences in the types of support you give each? Explain. Do you feel your support is appreciated? If so, how do you know? If not, why not?

2. Do you call on others for support or assistance when you need it? Why or why not? Is it appropriate to expect support from your co-workers and supervisors? Does reliance on the support of others make you dependent? What role should extended family play in supporting you with care issues?

3. What differences, if any, exist between the support given by men and women?

4. What is health? What is nutrition? What does it mean "to feel normal"?

5. Have you ever been given written instructions for health care to follow at home? Was this information helpful? If so, how? If not, why not?

6. Are Americans pill happy?

7. How is loneliness communicated?

8. Do racial and or ethnic groups view body image, health support, and responsibility for health care differently or similarly? Explain.

9. What impact, if any, has the dispersion of the family had on your ability to receive the support you needed?

10. Do the moods of others influence how you feel? How?

SUGGESTED READINGS

Social Support

Dressler, W. W. (1985). Extended family relationships, social support, and mental health in a southern black community. *Journal of Health & Social Behavior, 26*(1), 39–48.

Drummond, D. K. (2005). Diabetes management: An exploration into the verbal support attempts of relational others. *Qualitative Research Reports in Communication, 6*(1), 69–76.

Gleeson-Kreig, J., Bernal, H., & Woolley, S. (2002). The role of social support in the self-management of diabetes mellitus among a Hispanic population. *Public Health Nursing, 19*(3), 215–222.

Loneliness

Edwards, R. & Bello, R. (2001). The effects of loneliness and verbal aggressiveness on message interpretation. *Southern Communication Journal, 66*(2), 139–151.

Young-Ok, Y. & Clark, D. (2003). The relationships among loneliness, self/partner constructive maintenance behavior and relational satisfaction in two cultures. *Communication Studies, 54*(4), 451–467.

Pain Management

McDonald, D. D. & Molony, S. L. (2004). Postoperative pain communication skills for older adults. *Western Journal of Nursing Research, 26*(8), 836–852.

Telecommunications

Kenichi, I. (2006). Implications of mobility: The uses of personal communication media in everyday life. *Journal of Communication, 56*(2), 346–365.

5

Week Two Post-Surgery

TUESDAY, JUNE 3, 2003. One week since my surgery. Excitedly I jumped out of bed to prepare for the day, but something told me to call my doctor's office and verify the time of my appointment. When I called, the receptionist had no record of my appointment. She informed me that my doctor was off but would be in the next day. Frustrated, I didn't give up until she gave me a 2:45 p.m. appointment to see him. I immediately called Carol to see if she had left to pick me up. There was no answer and I left a message.

Carol, however, did not receive the message in time and knocked on my door at exactly 10:30 a.m. I opened the door and apologized profusely for not getting in touch with her in time for her to change her plans. Even though she assured me that she had been up for hours and out with her sons, I felt guilty for inconveniencing her. Carol said she would be happy to take me to my appointment the next day and asked, "Do you want to get out, get some movies, anything?" That is Carol for you . . . always helpful, always positive. Her eagerness to help me made me feel even worse. I couldn't wait to get her out of the apartment to alleviate my guilt. In my head I was screaming, "Please leave!" but with a smile on my face, I once again thanked her and tried to reassure her that I would not bother her again.

It rained off and on all day. It was as if Mother Earth was grounding me for wasting Carol's time. Homebound, I took a

shower for the first time post-surgery. There is nothing like a shower when you haven't had one in several days to make you feel 100 percent better! I secured my drain and incision area with plastic wrap and tape and enjoyed nearly 30 minutes of water pounding my body from head to toe. With squeaky-clean hair slapping me in the face, I stepped out of the shower, dried off, and redressed my incision area.

The apartment smelled like a sick room. I stripped the bed of its linens and spent the majority of the day doing laundry. Of course, while I did laundry Rana and Marlene called to check up on me. Rana was okay and had gotten the date of her appointment wrong. Her biopsy was actually the next day. As for nutrition, I got in 240 cc's of clear liquid, approximately 8 ounces, and 315 cc's of protein drink with 26 grams of protein. That is all I could manage. I had a cup to my mouth all day. Trying to get in the recommended nutrition is a lot of work and I found it much more tiring than doing laundry. Image . . . looking forward to loading and unloading the washing machine, folding and putting away clothes and linens . . . *an-ti-ci-pa-a-tion is making me wait*. Isn't that a song? I must be losing my mind! Before falling asleep I left a message on Jeanne's voice mail asking for a ride to my doctor's appointment.

I *really* do not like being dependent on other people.

WEDNESDAY, JUNE 4, 2003. Irritated that I hadn't heard from Jeanne, I looked through my closet for an outfit that would be comfortable and nonbinding especially around my abdomen. I chose a long straight-line, pin-stripped, shirt dress, sandals, and scarf. After pressing the dress, I called Cheryl E. and asked her for a ride to my appointment.

"I won't be able to take you because I have a 3:00 p.m. meeting on HIV, but I'll ask my secretary to give you a ride." she said. "You will really like her!"

"No, I don't feel comfortable with that. I will just ask one of my co-workers. Thanks."

"Well, if your co-worker doesn't work out, please let me know."

"I will," I responded, hung up, and immediately called Carol L. and left a message on her voice mail requesting assistance. *Damn, I really do not like asking my co-workers to do things for me! I wonder if they think I don't have any friends who care enough to help me. I do not like being dependent on other people!*

I left messages with Carol L., Cheryl E., Shawn, and Jeanne asking for a lift to my doctor's appointment . . . four messages! By 11:30 a.m. I hadn't heard from any of them. *How will I get to my appointment?* My sister was off and I called her home in Conover. No answer. I wasn't surprised; she was probably getting ready for the AME district conference. Anyway, it would upset her to know that I don't have a ride. I didn't leave a message. She would feel obligated to come. Is it fair to ask her to drive 45 minutes out of her way to take me somewhere when she has her own family to take care of? Is such a request appropriate when I know her daughter is having a tonsillectomy tomorrow? *I absolutely hate being dependent on others! I must get this drain out so I can get around by myself!*

Okay, let's try someone else. I called Cheryl S. She had just gotten back in town after vacationing in Florida and was distressed to hear that I had major surgery while she was gone. She was not available to assist me, however, because of plans and commitments already made. We spent the rest of the conversation engaged in small talk and ended with her promise to call later to see how my appointment went and arrange a get-together for later in the week.

I am really beginning to think that my social support network isn't worth two cents. Maybe I'm being punished for my selfishness throughout the years. Can I drive myself to this appointment? What do I do with this drain? How can I wear a seatbelt with this drain in? Will driving 20 to 25 minutes one way tire me out? What dangers could result from such an act? I know this, if no one steps up to assist me before 2:00 p.m., I will drive myself! People are busy these days with their own problems and needs. Maybe it is unrealistic to expect anyone to be there for me. I feel alone. Oh

God, I feel helpless and I feel like I'm begging people to pay attention to me and my problems! I don't like this feeling!

A girl's gotta do what a girl's gotta do. Amen!

I showered, redressed my incision, brushed my teeth, dressed and drove myself to my appointment. Twenty minutes later I was in my surgeon's office signing in.

Once again, the receptionist did not have a record of my appointment. She, however, instructed me to sit down and she would make sure the doctor saw me. Within 25 minutes I was called back and weighed. My weight was 235 lbs. I had lost 11 pounds if you went by my doctor's scale and 13 pounds by my home scale. A nurse escorted me into one of the examination rooms and instructed me to get on top of the examination table. Once I was on the table, she unbuttoned the area around my abdomen, exposing the incisions. Dr. Bozeman walked in, full of humor and obviously in an good mood.

"Hello, Dr. Drummond. I'm going to remove the drain. You will feel a funny sensation, but it shouldn't hurt."

This was the first time he called me "doctor," and I must admit that I liked the acknowledgment. As he held firmly and pulled, I could feel the ¼-inch-round tube retreating through my intestine and stomach. He was right; it didn't hurt. The nurse removed the staples from the other five sites on my abdomen and bandaged them. She instructed me not to remove the tape and to let it work itself free. Then she covered the area where the drain had been removed with gauze.

"There will probably still be drainage in this area so you will have to replace the gauze frequently. Don't forget to cover this area when showering," she reminded me. You don't want to get this area wet until the incision has closed."

"Dr. Bozeman," I asked, "have any of your patients complained or mentioned vision changes?"

He looked closely at my face and behind my ears and said, "Your vision is affected by the Transderm Scop patch you have behind your ear. Remove it. You shouldn't need the patches anymore."

I removed the patch immediately, and said, "A friend of mine knows one of your former patients. She told my friend that she wants to discuss depression with me."

"No! I don't want you to get caught up in talking about depression! Every patient is different, and more than likely you won't experience depression at all. Each individual's experience is as different as her anatomy."

"Have you read any of the journals of your patients?"

"No, primarily because I do not get involved with all the support group stuff. It would take too much time to read the journals."

He asked for a report on my protein and liquid intake, encouraged me to make my own protein drinks to get the maximum level of protein in the least amount of liquid, and instructed me to take a children's chewable multivitamin for the next month.

"I really do not know how much liquid my pouch is capable of holding," I said, "and I am really afraid to test it to see."

"Good, we have trained you well. We do not want you to test the capacity of the pouch."

Satisfied, I asked, "Do I need to continue taking that anti-hypertension drug, Diovan?"

He spoke quietly to the nurse for a minute, who then took my blood pressure. She told him that my blood pressure was 112/60. He turned toward me and said, "You do not need this medication anymore. Please discuss everything that has happened with your family physician because anti-hypertension drugs can cause severe side effects to the liver and kidney if stopped abruptly. Everything looks good so I will not need to see you again for at least 3 weeks. Make sure you keep your June 10 appointment with the nutritionist. You don't have to stop at the front desk. There is no charge for this visit."

I thanked the doctor and nurse and headed out. As I left, I felt free! I slowly breathed in and exhaled that clean Carolina air. It was as if I had been injected with an infusion of energy and warmth. My body felt fresh and new and I couldn't help but laugh and smile

to myself. I was truly on top of the world . . . at least on top of crushing that Diovan! What a relief to not have to take that pill again! I hate pills! On top of that, I wouldn't have to look at or deal with that drain anymore as a constant reminder of surgery and dependence on others! At that moment I knew that everything would be okay and that I could now take care of myself.

On the drive back to Charlotte I stopped at a gas station and filled the tank. All I wanted was to return home and call my friends to share my good news. Upon entering the apartment, I immediately checked voice mail to see if my pleas for help made earlier that day had been returned. No. Not one message. I shrugged off my disappointment, went to my home office, and began to edit a paper. I had no problems with my vision.

Getting healthy and staying healthy through a focus on good nutrition is extremely difficult. Once again I attempted to get more liquid in my system from one hour to the next. True, I did a little better than the day before, but not much better. I got in 360 cc's of protein drink with 28 grams of protein and 240 cc's of clear liquid. I was considering Dr. Bozeman's suggestion that I buy protein powder and make my own more concentrated drinks.

THURSDAY, JUNE 5, 2003. I felt energetic and decided to go into the office and work on my research and new classes for the fall. After packing two cans of Ensure, as well as bottled water and Crystal Light into a canvas bag, I showered, dressed, and drove to campus. Once there, I talked with our administrative assistant for a little while. She commented that I looked as if I had lost some weight. I didn't respond, because I was not ready to share with her how I was losing the weight.

I love libraries and will use any excuse to visit one, including returning books even when I do not plan to check out more. Five books were overdue and I reasoned the exercise would be good for me. My walk to the library took nearly 20 minutes from the office and back. When I returned to my office, I went through all of the e-mail I received for the past week and came across a message

from my department chair. It stated, "I hope you are recovering well; I am sorry I could not do more to help you find transportation this morning. Do let me know if you need anything." That was thoughtful. In addition, he took the time to stop in my office and let me know I was in his thoughts and if I needed anything, to just ask. I felt the sincerity. Sometimes all you need to feel better is an acknowledgment of what you are going through from someone else. They don't have to *do* a thing.

In the hallway, I ran into Carol, who exclaimed excitedly, "You have lost weight! That dress looks loose on you now!"

"Yes, I have lost between 10 and 13 pounds!"

"Do you crave texture, like chicken nuggets, since you haven't had anything but liquids?"

"No, not really, I don't think about solid foods because I know I can't have them. So what is the point of obsessing about them?"

We briefly discussed my recent visit to the doctor to have the drain removed and then she asked, "Does anyone else in the department know about your surgery? If not, you don't need to worry that they will find out from me."

"No, no one else knows, and I don't think I'm ready to discuss it with any of them yet. Of course, Shawn knows I had surgery, but I think he thinks it is just a woman's thing and hasn't asked any specifics. Thanks, I really appreciate your discretion."

I returned to my office and tried to work. I could not, however, stop thinking about bowel movements. After my surgery and during my hospital stay I had a bowel movement that was watery and diarrhea-like. Its coloring was the darkest brown, almost black. Since leaving the hospital, my movements were still watery but the color was consistently light to medium brown. It seems strange to pay so much attention to one's excrement, but I've become more and more sensitive and in tune to what is happening in my body. Plus, I think I heard somewhere that your excrement is a good indicator of your health. I wonder, what is my shit trying to tell me about my health? Right now, it is definitely telling me there hasn't

been a morsel of solid food in this body for a while! I worked a few more hours until I got tired and decided to return home.

At home, I slipped into bed and watched television. As I lay, I noticed three small white birds perched upon my balcony. I had not seen white birds this close before. They sat there facing my French doors. I slowly got out of bed and walked toward the door expecting the birds to fly away. I reached the door and stared at them. They did not fly away. They looked at me as I looked at them. They all had pink feet and one had a light-blue tab wrapped around one leg. I felt overwhelming peace, as I felt like my mother was with me, supporting me and approving of my actions. As the birds flew away, I opened the door, walked out onto the balcony and looked out beyond the trees. I cried tears of joy for the love of my mother and tears of sadness for the intense loneliness I now felt.

FRIDAY, JUNE 06, 2003. The phone rang and it was Amy from my nutritionist's office. She said, "I bet you can't wait to eat some real food! Well, you can start on Tuesday! We will see you at 7:30 a.m. Bye!"

I took my medications Levaquin, Prevacid, and Carafate, dressed, and got my things together for work, then drove to the nearest grocery store. In the GNC section, I spent quite some time examining and reading all of the labels on the various protein powders. It was overwhelming. Luckily, the store manager, a 30-something African American woman, helped me decide which product to purchase. My choices included powders with 17 grams of protein to those with 40 grams of protein per scoop. The containers were huge and expensive, ranging from $28 to $40. I bought a product called Optimum Nutrition 100% Whey Protein Dietary Supplement with 22 grams of protein per scoop, as well as a chewable multivitamin designed for children.

The store manager approved of my protein supplement selection. She said she did not drink milk and would mix her protein powder with water and two scoops of whipped cream to make it taste as good as a milkshake or malt. It occurred to me that my

nutritionist would probably have a problem with the fat and sugar components of whipped cream and prefer that I use skim milk. At my next appointment, I would ask if she had any recipes for protein shakes.

Upon arriving on campus, I shared my surgery experience with my colleague and friend Jon. Jon has an aunt who was over 400 pounds before she had weight-loss surgery. He seemed to understand the seriousness of our decision to have the surgery and complimented me for tackling my health issues in addition to coping with the death of my mother and all of the stress entailed in being a tenure-track professor. We discussed his latest horror project and students, then I went to my office to work.

"Are you going to tell me what's going on now?" asked another colleague, Cheryl Spainhour, as she stood in the doorway of my office. I told her about my diagnoses with Type II diabetes, hypertension, gastric reflux disease, sleep apnea, and thyroid problems and that the quickest fix was gastric bypass surgery. When I mentioned "gastric bypass surgery," she did not know or understand to what I was referring.

"You know, the surgery Al Roker and Carnie Wilson had to lose weight!" I said emphatically, finding it hard to believe that she didn't know what I was talking about! As it finally dawned on her what I had done, she sat back in the chair holding her stomach with her mouth open in shock. She wanted to know why I had kept this secret and seemed disappointed that I had not talked to her about my situation earlier. As she calmed down, we discussed the department politics, our fall classes, and the children's book she was writing, then made plans to get together to go to our favorite bookstores and theaters before the end of summer.

"I can't wait to have scrambled eggs and grits next week and to go out to lunch once I can eat solid food again!" I groaned as I slumped across my desk.

"We don't have to do anything around food. In fact, I am not going to bring up the topic of food," Cheryl said, assuring me that

she was in my corner and that I could call on her anytime for anything. An enthusiastic teacher of journalism, she remembered one of her students wrote a fairly humorous article about gastric bypass surgery. She promised to find a copy of it for me.

After speaking with Cheryl, I went to the Chair's office and talked with him about publishing companies, the differences between university presses and textbook publishers, and the status of various academic journals. When I returned to my office, Cindy was waiting outside my door. She has been going through a lot lately with the separation from her husband and taking on the role of a single parent to a teenage daughter. For the last several months, I've noticed that she has lost a great deal of weight. She claims she has been less interested in eating out and much more conscious of her eating habits since leaving her husband. I complimented her weight lost but did not tell her about my surgery. I'm not sure why. Maybe I had discussed it enough for one day. I didn't think she would be judgmental, but it felt wrong to talk about weight-loss surgery with someone who was successfully losing weight by simply changing her eating habits.

At Target, I purchased a Hamilton Beach Drink Master because it is small and designed especially for mixing drinks. I knew I wanted something that would look good on my kitchen countertop next to my black coffee maker and my three-quart ice-tea maker. I would use it only to mix my protein drinks. The silver container has a 4-ounce mark that makes it easier to mix exactly 4 ounces of skim milk with one scoop of the protein powder. I would obtain my daily protein requirement in just 8 ounces of liquid, which is much more manageable than trying to drink 36 to 48 ounces of Ensure, Boost, or Kashi Go-Lean throughout the day.

When I got home, I mixed a scoop of protein with 4 ounces of skim milk, poured 2 ounces into a glass, and took 15 to 20 minutes to savor it. It wasn't any less tasty than the Ensure, Boost, or Go-Lean. The more it sat and the more I realized I would be getting in 32 grams of protein, the better it tasted.

Shawn phoned to make sure I was okay and asked if I needed anything. I told him that I was fine and had been in the office the past 2 days. He told me he would be in Charlotte the entire weekend if I needed anything. It was good to know he cares. But what happened to Jeanne and Cheryl E., my so-called sisters? Why hadn't they returned my calls?

It was a quiet weekend. Streets flooded as the rain pounded the city, forcing me to remain inside. Just sitting around, however, didn't appeal to me. I did housework—washing clothes and ironing. I even ironed things that I couldn't get into, in anticipation of the moment when I could. My closet contained sizes 14 through 28, so I wouldn't need to buy any clothes anytime soon.

On Sunday mornings, I usually call my brother Tim, who lives nearly 3 hours away. When I called this morning, his wife, Virginia, answered. We made tentative plans for me to visit them before the summer ended before she turned the phone over to Tim. We talked about the usual things, teaching as a thankless profession, lack of funds to survive the summer, our plans for the upcoming academic year, current events, especially foreign affairs, and then he asked, "How is the diabetes?"

"Cured, I no longer have diabetes. I had surgery, bariatric surgery, 2 weeks ago. When I walked out of the hospital, my blood sugar was 94 and my blood pressure was 112/60. I don't have to take any of the medications I was taking before, including the medications for my diabetes, Glucotrol, and Glucophague, and the anti-hypertensive, Diovan. I lost 13 pounds in the first week and expect to be down approximately 40 pounds by July. I apologize for not telling you about my plans to have surgery, but I did not want to worry you, and frankly I did not want anyone to discourage me from having the surgery."

Tim did not seem upset by this news. I suspected Marlene had already told him about the surgery since he had spoken with her last weekend and she hadn't mentioned the conversation to me. "Excellent, you are an adult and capable of making your own

decisions," he said. "I think it was the right decision given your similarity to Mom. You are the most like her and it was probably a good thing to address the diabetes as soon as possible . . . Wow, you have inspired me to go and work out. So, when I see you, I will not recognize you!"

My only brother was diagnosed with Type II diabetes when he was in his 30s. I always thought this unusual because he is in relatively good shape. He exercises regularly and is always within 5 to 20 pounds of his ideal weight. Marlene and I do not understand how this happened to him. For me, it just confirms the role of heredity in illness experience.

"How is *your* diabetes?" I asked.

"My doctor says I need to lose 5 more pounds. My ideal weight is 195, and my goal is to get off of the Glucotrol as soon as possible."

I interrupted him with, "You know, I really believe that taking those drugs for years actually causes damage to your kidneys and liver. I don't think they make that clear. If they did, I think most people would make changes sooner. I know I don't want to end up on a dialysis machine!"

He replied, "I agree they have to affect the kidneys and liver. That is why I am determined to stop them as soon as possible. Wow, you have really inspired me to work out today!"

We talked about protein powders and multivitamins and agreed that they are the key to more energy. He uses a powder to get 50 grams of protein a day and drinks a lot of Gatorade to rehydrate. I admired his determination and all the work he puts into exercising and hoped it would be contagious. I wanted exercise to become my daily desire. I want to crave it as I used to crave potatoes!

Both my sister and brother seem to understand why I've done this. They are my life. They are all I have left of my mother, and their approval means everything to me.

After speaking with my brother, I couldn't help but think about food. I wanted scrabbled eggs and grits so badly I could taste

them! Don't get me wrong, I wasn't hungry. I just wanted a different taste, a different texture in my mouth. Protein drinks come in a limited number of flavors and I was tired of them. I was tired of looking for new recipes and trying new ingredients to mix together to get the taste of a milkshake. No matter what I do, I haven't been able to achieve that. I couldn't stop looking at the list of soft foods I could eat beginning Tuesday. Tuna, mashed potatoes, toast, and applesauce dominated my thoughts. The list included baby foods, yogurt, and cottage cheese, but I wasn't interested in those foods. What else could I have? I couldn't wait to see the nutritionist on Tuesday and get a more complete list.

MONDAY, MONDAY! JUNE 9, 2003. I felt weak. I took a multivitamin, Prevacid, and Carafate with a few sips of water, removed the bandages from my incision area and took a long shower. Still tired, I thought an increase in water or protein would make me feel better. I drank 60 cc's of Ensure as I sat in front of the television and listened to Matt Lauer discuss a special tribute to Luther Vandross that Tamira Gray, a former *American Idol* contestant, would be doing on *The Today Show* the next day.

Luther Vandross lives and is apparently about to die with diabetes. Luther, was it a stroke or heart attack that landed you in the hospital? I can't remember. Does it really matter? So many complications result from living with diabetes that you could die of anything. The fact is that he was overweight for most of his life, tried to lose weight through one diet program or another, and succeeded as evidenced by his album covers, but still wound up fighting for his life.

No, that will not happen to me! I packed a bag with cans of Ensure and water, grabbed my laptop and folders and headed out the door. I walked down three flights of stairs, got into my car, and drove to campus. By the time I got to the office, I was panting and sweating profusely and had to sit down to rest. But my thirst was quenched with water and my body energized with Ensure. I felt better and worked with the music of Luther Vandross playing softly in the background. After a couple of hours, I decided to take a

break and go to the library to return several books received through interlibrary loan, avoiding the $1 per day late fee for each book. I put the books into a canvas bag, packed some bottled water, and made my way to the elevator.

In the elevator headed down to the first floor, I convinced myself that walking the 10 minutes to the library would be good for me. Since it was hot outside, *very* hot and approaching 80 degrees, I walked slowly, so slowly that I wondered if others noticed. As I inched along, I looked into the faces of those I passed, hoping they could not see the fear of fainting in my eyes. The canvas bag, which held the books I sought to return, was heavy. I switched the bag from hand to hand in an attempt to make its load feel lighter. The sun beat down upon me and I could feel a light spray of sweat on my face.

When I made it to the circulation desk located near the entrance to the library, I slowly removed each book from the bag and waited as the librarian recorded the return date on each. She finished and I quickly exited the library, gulped from my water bottle, and placed my hand across my mouth as I gagged. The walk back to my office was just as slow as my walk to the library but not as tiring. I had had enough for one day and packed up my laptop and papers. Five minutes and two flights of stairs later, I was at my car in the faculty parking lot. I had to return to my office, however, to retrieve my wallet that I had locked in my office desk.

Back at the complex, I got my mail from the mail center, parked my car in its usual space, grabbed my laptop and canvas bag, and ascended the three flights of stairs to my home. I rested at both the second and third floor landings. It felt good to be home again. My sister was calling every day to check on my progress. This was no different. She had no idea how much this meant to me. Sometimes I feel as if I go for days without speaking to another human being. I just hope I don't become so dependent on her and then I lose her like I did our mother. I don't know how I would survive. As I tossed and turned throughout the night, I thought about food and the good news I hoped to hear from my nutritionist.

DISCUSSION QUESTIONS

1. What do the terms *health* and *normal* mean to you? What are the various approaches to health taken by health-care professionals? How are these approaches learned? Is one better than another? What aspects of a person's communication behavior denote the philosophical stance he or she has on health?

2. Do you want your doctor to be emotionally involved or in tune with you? Why or why not? What are the rewards or consequences for health professionals who are emotionally attached to their patients?

3. Have you talked openly with friends, coworkers, or acquaintances about any medical procedures you have had? Are there some procedures that are more open to discussion then others? Why? What purpose does secrecy serve?

SUGGESTED READINGS

Apker, J. (2005). Role negotiation, stress, and burnout: A day in the life of "supernurse." In E. B. Ray (Ed.), *Health communication in practice: A case study approach* (pp. 245–260). Mahwah, NY: Lawrence Erlbaum Associates.

Barnes, M. K., & Duck, S. (1994). Everyday communicative contexts for social support. In B. R. Burleson, T. L. Albrecht, & I. G. Sarason (Eds.), *Communication of social support: Messages, interactions, relationships, and community* (pp. 175–194). Thousand Oaks, CA: Sage.

Du Pré, A. (2005). Making empowerment work: Medical center soars in satisfaction ratings. In E. B. Ray (Ed.), *Health communication in practice: A case study approach* (pp. 311–322). Mahwah, NY: Lawrence Erlbaum Associates.

Novack, D. H., Suchman, A. L., Clark, W., Epstein, R. M., Najberg, G. E., & Kaplan, C. (1997). Calibrating the physician:

Personal awareness and effective patient care. *Journal of the American Medical Association, 278,* 502–510.

Zook, E. G. (1993). Embodied health and constitutive communication: Toward an authentic conceptualization of health communication. *Communication Yearbook, 17,* 344–377.

6

Week Three Post-Surgery

A New Focus on Nutrition

TUESDAY, JUNE 10, 2003—finally here! The day I can have some real food, and even though it has to be as soft as baby food, I can't wait! I am not hungry, but I just can't stand the taste or feel of another protein shake in my mouth.

I got out of bed, took my Carafate, Prevacid, and multivitamin, showered, dressed, and drove the 15 to 20 minutes to Concord to the Diabetes Management Center to see my nutritionist, Dee Short, RN. The Center is located on the lefthand side of the street across from the entrance to the hospital and only a block from my surgeon's office. Everyone on my health-care team is conveniently located and accessible.

At 7:35 a.m. Amy escorted me back to Dee's office and directed me to get on the scale, which registered 228 pounds—20 pounds fewer than before surgery! Dee congratulated me and said that they expect individuals to lose anywhere between 10 and 25 pounds within 2 weeks. Generally, individuals who have more to lose—those over 300 pounds—lose the most. She was impressed that someone under 250 pounds had lost so much in the first 2 weeks. I credited the walking and getting out of the house as soon as possible for this.

Dee's desk was overflowing with food products, and her wall was covered with the pictures of her clients at various weights,

announcing their successful weight loss. She took my blood pressure, which was 124/60, and apologized for not having a working meter to take my blood sugar. After viewing my hospital records, she indicated that I shouldn't have a problem, but to be on the safe side, I should check my blood sugar once a week for a month just to make sure. She assured me that she would be ready to measure my blood sugar during my next appointment.

She asked if the nurses at the hospital had discussed the "insulin protocol" with me before I left. I stated that they hadn't but a nurse at my endocrinologist's office had before surgery. She said this was an issue that they had been trying to address for a while. Apparently since one of my illnesses presurgery was diabetes, the floor nurses at the hospital were supposed to test me to see if I remembered what my endocrinology nurse had taught me . . . that I was to take insulin if my blood sugar went over 160 or under 75. Intuitively I knew that this wasn't a concern because I hadn't experienced any signs or symptoms of high or low blood sugar since my discharge.

My nutritionist is a registered nurse, which gives me peace of mind. She got right down to business and presented me with a handout entitled "2 Week Post Op Nutrition Plan," which she explained in detail.

"The most important thing for you to do is to get in the necessary protein and drink water to avoid dehydration," she said.

"Can I eat an egg with grits?"

"Because you can only eat 2 ounces, you wouldn't be able to eat both in one meal."

I was disappointed but understood.

"However, you can increase the protein value of the grits by cooking them in skim milk instead of water. Your diet for the next week should consist exclusively of grits, oatmeal, cream of wheat, protein soups, eggs, cottage cheese, yogurt, skim milk, light crackers, whole wheat bread, mozzarella string cheese, and beans, all types of beans including pintos, black, black-eyed peas, kidney

beans, and fat-free refried beans. Of course, you can still have a smoothie made with protein powder, yogurt, skim milk, and fruit, specifically, bananas or strawberries."

"According to the paperwork given me when I was discharged from the hospital, I can also have baby foods, including meats, tuna, and mashed potatoes," I added.

"Disregard the papers from the hospital and any other nutritional information given you by Dr. Bozeman or anyone else. You are under a 'diabetes protocol.' Since diabetes runs rampant in your family and I know you want to avoid getting diabetes again, you need to avoid starches now! No potatoes, no potatoes, no potatoes!"

The potato . . . I had had a love affair with the potato since birth! I had eaten the potato in some form every day since I was 17 and in college. Not every other day. *Every day.* Fried, baked, mashed, boiled, or scalloped. But guess what people? It is a new day, and yes, *yes, I am willing to give up the potato to save my life!* This is big! This is huge! This is what I must do and I know it! I will change and give up the potato!

Dee continued, "You should avoid using sweet pickles in your tuna, use dill instead, and avoid applesauce. These things could cause you to experience the 'dumping syndrome.' This is the most violent form of diarrhea one can ever experience, and believe me if you go through it once you will never, ever want to experience it again!"

She talked about the things I could eat and how to prepare them for maximum taste and protein as she pointed to them on her desk. The handout outlined the foods and vitamins I would need for the fourth, fifth, and sixth weeks post-surgery. In the margins of the handout, she wrote the dates I could start each significant change in diet. In the fourth week I noted that I could have fish and would begin taking calcium and complex B vitamins. It wouldn't be until the fifth week that I could have chicken and turkey and the sixth before I could begin eating lean red meats, pork, and ham with a couple of tablespoons of vegetables or fruit.

"You will lose weight doing absolutely nothing, but you will maximize your weight loss by walking as much as possible," Dee said. "Your nutritional management plan includes a personal trainer to assist you in designing a lifelong exercise program. Here is his name and phone number. Please contact him in the sixth week post-op."

Then, to end our meeting, we set up appointments for the next three months.

Afterwards, I bought grits, four varieties of Fanatic high-protein soups, peanut butter, a six-pack of bottled water, string mozzarella, whole-wheat bread, eggs, and Dannon light yogurt, and spent a total of $27.16. I have never had cottage cheese, yogurt, and most of the beans, and I was concerned that I may not like enough of the foods to survive. Nevertheless, the realization hit me that my food bills would be drastically less than what I usually spent. Even though single, I generally spent $40 to $80 a week on groceries. Those groceries included the best grade of steaks, chicken, bacon, sausage, and other pork products. I spent a lot of money on fresh vegetables and never bargain-shopped when it came to food, never used coupons, and always went for the best brands.

As Dee suggested, I began to keep a record of my daily consumption. My first record reads as follows: At breakfast (9:30 a.m.) I had one large scrambled egg with ½ slice of reduced-fat American cheese and skim milk, consisting of 11 grams of protein. I wasn't able to eat the whole egg, because I felt it moving back up my esophagus and realized my pouch was *already* full! I had always loved scrambled eggs, but my taste was changing because I had to fight to eat the little I did. Even with cheese, pepper, and garlic powder, the egg tasted bland. At 11:00 a.m. I had a snack: 2 ounces of skim milk, providing me with another 2 grams of protein. Two hours later for lunch I made a smoothie with 2 ounces of skim milk, 2 ounces of yogurt and one scoop of protein powder for a total of 26 grams of protein. My second snack of the day at 5:00 p.m., worth only 1 gram of protein, consisted of ¼ slice of

whole-wheat bread with American cheese. I really enjoyed the toast! Then for dinner I tried my first protein soup, called Cha Cha Chili. Of course, I could have only 2 ounces and topped it with one mozzarella stick for flavor and a total of 10 grams of protein. Before bed I had 2 ounces of yogurt to add another 2 grams of protein to my total for the day. By the end of the day, I had managed to consume enough food to get a total of 52 grams of protein, and felt really energized!

Support Group Drama

Many of Dr. Bozeman's patients attend a support group meeting conducted by our nutritionist, Dee, on the first Tuesday of each month at 6:00 p.m. As a scholar, I am interested in the concept of social support and was excited to attend my first meeting as a patient. The group meets at the Medical Arts Center at NEMC in a classroom beneath the cafeteria across from the theater area.

Upon entering the classroom I saw five to six women between the ages of 55 and 65 sitting at a couple of tables. The room was large with 30 to 40 medium-size tables that could seat two to three individuals, a podium, and chalkboards. I approached the women and asked, "Is this where the bariatric support group meets?"

"Yes!" they sang out in unison. One laughingly commented, "I guess you couldn't tell since none of us are fat, huh?"

"That's right," I replied with a smile and sat down at a table behind them. One of the women rose, leaned across the table, and handed me a sign-in notebook. The sign-in sheet requested your name and surgery date. Some of the women had had their surgeries nearly a year before. I signed the book, passed it on, and waited for the session to begin. Others filled the room but only three men were present out of the nearly 40 to 45 individuals that came. I thought this was a large number for a support group but remembered Dee saying in a previous conversation that she preferred large groups over smaller ones of 6 to 8 individuals.

I sat alone until a large 400- to 500-pound gentleman took the seat beside me. He smelled. Yes, I could smell him. It wasn't entirely an unpleasant smell but a mixture of cologne and body musk, a strong smell that violently assaulted my nose. He introduced himself and immediately announced that he was having the surgery that Friday. The smell made it hard for me to concentrate on what he was saying and I missed his name. Despite this, I introduced myself and informed him that I had the surgery 2 weeks before.

"How much weight have you lost?" he asked. He seemed surprised yet excited at my 20-pound loss and continued to ask me questions as the meeting progressed. Once Dee, the group facilitator, arrived she walked around the room and greeted people while handing out two circulars. One sheet was entitled "Behavior Modification," and the other delineated good food sources with the vitamins and minerals contained in each. The Behavior Modification sheet discussed forming good eating habits, reiterating ideas we've all heard before — don't eat in front of the television, or while reading, cooking, or feeling angry. New habits should include eating on a small, decorative plate, eating three meals a day and two snacks, eating slowly, serving from the stove instead of family-style, and leaving food on your plate.

When Dee finally started the meeting she wanted to know who needed diet request cards for local restaurants. I raised my hand since I didn't have any. She let us know that we could get others from Dr. Bozeman. The card basically announces the surgical weight management program of the hospital with the nutritionist name on one side. The other side was labeled, "special diet request." Then there was a blank for the patient to sign his or her name. After the blank read the following, "The above named person has had surgery to reduce the stomach to 3 ounces. Please allow this person to order a smaller portion or senior citizen portion. Thank you." Beneath the statement is the nutritionist's signature. I thought . . . *this will come in handy when I am ready to eat out*

even though that will be months away. But do I really want people to know
that I had the surgery? I probably won't use these but, just in case, I'll
keep some.

Dee made it clear that these support meetings were designed
for those who had already had the surgery but noted that there
were six or seven individuals present who were scheduled to have
it in the next few months. After handing out the cards, she asked
those who had the surgery to introduce themselves and to give
their surgery date and amount of weight loss. The women had
weight losses ranging from 17 to 160 pounds, and their surgery
dates ranged from that past Wednesday to those who had it a year
earlier. The woman who had the surgery a year earlier passed
around pictures of herself at her present weight in clothes at her
largest weight. Impressive! She was truly half the woman she was
previously! Sadly, she said that she wished she had kept a record of
her measurements so she could tell us how many inches she lost.
Once everyone introduced themselves, Dee announced that as a
group we represented 1,400 lost pounds! Wow! Then, she opened
the floor up for questions and comments.

It struck me as I sat there that I was the only African American. I was the only person of color and I was probably one of the
youngest there. These were white women and men between the
ages of 55 and 70 with maybe three or four individuals in their
mid-30s. But that's it! I really wanted to talk with a black woman
in her 40s who had had the surgery. Was this an unrealistic expec-
tation? How many black women have even had this surgery who
live in North Carolina, on the East Coast, or in this country? Why
does this even matter to me? Disappointed, I remained to listen
and see what I could learn from those present. Though most
ignored me (and I must admit that I am not the most outgoing
person), several made me feel welcomed, especially the young
man who sat next to me.

The meeting was enlightening, to say the least. I was surprised
at how many admitted to inappropriate behavior that ended with

them spending additional time in the hospital. One woman admitted to eating noodles during her first week post-surgery and damaging her pouch, which had barely began the healing process. She had to return to the hospital. Another woman was fixing lunch for her kids and forgot about the strict nutritional guidelines she was instructed to follow and ended up eating a hot dog! She ended up in the hospital, too. Several talked about overeating and stretching their pouches! One woman talked about not drinking water for days after her surgery, breaking out into rashes, and getting a bladder infection that required her to take additional medications.

As tale after ghastly tale was shared, it began to sink into my hard head that I was truly one of the blessed. I had no equally appalling story to tell! My audacity to silently question my surgeon's insistence that I keep a drain in for 1 week after surgery melted away as another woman talked about her experience postop when she did not have a drain and ended up spending 3 additional months in the hospital! I would put up with 2 to 3 weeks of a drain to avoid going back behind those walls!

Many admitted to not exercising at all. I was shocked! I would think that exercise would be a must to tone up the body. That did explain why many of them did not look toned. Most of the discussion focused on the need for cosmetic surgery to handle redundant skin. This was news to me, and having read everything that I could get my hands on about gastric bypass surgery, I was surprised that I hadn't read anything about this concern. Dee stated that at least 4 out of the nearly 400 patients that she had supervised in the last 2 years had some type of cosmetic surgery and that many of us would probably need some form of this surgery. Dr. Bozeman and others were working to get health insurance plans to pay for it. Only one client had been able to get her insurance company to pay for her cosmetic surgery. One woman had gotten her breasts lifted and 10 inches of skin removed from them. Another had her tummy tucked, her breasts lifted, and her underarms done. According to Dee, many patients have to pay out of pocket, and the cost may be

high. For example, to get rid of the skin underneath the upper arm area is approximately $2,700.

Several obviously frustrated individuals complained that Dr. Bozeman had turned them down for the gastric bypass surgery. All were over 400 pounds and had assumed that their weight alone would get them on the operation table. They were shocked to find out that they would have to lose 50 pounds or more using traditional methods before the surgeon would even talk to them. Dee pointed out that many doctors do not like to do surgery on extremely obese people because their livers tend to have a lot of fat around them, which can complicate surgery.

"Then he needs to put that information on his Web site!" exclaimed one of the denied individuals.

Another added, "I tried to get Dr. Bozeman to do my surgery for months and he turned me down. He said it was too risky because I had two open-heart surgeries, experienced complications from my diabetes including a problem with my eyes that required surgery, was diagnosed with thyroid cancer, have knee problems requiring surgery, and other problems I don't care to mention. I found another surgeon who agreed to do my bariatric surgery! This surgeon in Charlotte, Dr. Block, did a less invasive surgery on me, a banded one. I'm glad, but I've only lost 21 pounds in 5 weeks."

These comments led to a discussion about the pros and cons of different types of bariatric surgery. All I heard was that one generally achieves much more weight loss with the bypass surgery.

Much of the discussion centered on quality-of-life issues. An older woman exclaimed excitedly that the greatest benefit from the surgery for her was an increase in her sexual activity. Everyone laughed. They talked about increased opportunities to date, the ability to sit at booths in restaurants, play with grandchildren, go back to work, and shop in regular clothing stores. One woman commented that shopping and trying on clothes had become her number-one pastime. She would go into stores and try on lots of

clothes with no intention of buying anything. A couple of the women brought with them the clothes they outgrew to share with others and agreed to take the clothes that no one wanted to Goodwill. They suggested everyone shop at value or thrift stores for the things they needed to avoid spending a great deal of money on clothes that would be too big in less than a month.

Even though this talk aroused my expectations, I was surprised that no one mentioned any health benefits such as ridding themselves of diabetes, hypertension, and a variety of other ailments, and the money they saved by no longer having to pay for the medications to manage them. These are the benefits I see! Am I weird? No. These are white people. For many white people, it seems to me, weight management seems to be all about body image! And for African Americans it seems to be all about improving health. We all are probably concerned about both but tend to see one as more important than the other. In the end, I think, we all need to get on the health bandwagon.

The talk soon turned to hunger, diet, and food choices, particularly the best protein powders and smoothie recipes. There was a great deal of talk about being hungry, and I was surprised at how some had been hungry the day after surgery and felt as if they were starving during the first 2 weeks post-op. To curb their hunger they chewed gum. The doctors and nutritionist, however, advised us *not* to chew gum. Swallowing gum may damage the pouch, and at least one person admitted to having such problems. Chewing gum produces saliva in the mouth, which makes one feel better, but it may also lead to more production of acid in the stomach, which is not a good thing.

The young man sitting next to me asked if it were true that one can never take medications again after having gastric bypass surgery. He wanted to know if it was impossible to swallow a pill or vitamin. Others quickly dispelled this myth by enumerating the vitamins and medicines they take and informed him that "pills are taken with just a sip of water." They gave advice on how to handle

constipation, diarrhea, and back pain. Many experienced back pain after losing 50 or more pounds. In overweight individuals, the lower disk in one's back may compress, and as one loses weight the disk becomes less compressed but may be already damaged from years of handling too much weight. Those with this problem had surgery to correct the compression or took medications to handle the pain.

Doubts and fears about having the surgery on the actual day of surgery were expressed. One woman claimed that she told her husband to take her back home once they reached the hospital and once home made him go back. Nearly everyone seemed to think this was "normal." I never had a doubt—not one! I remember being excited the day of surgery and wanting it to be over so I could start changing my life. If I had a fear it was that some reason such as a cold would be found to prevent the surgery from taking place that day. Does that make me "abnormal" or just "different?" *Different,* I decided. I am just different.

A praise session began. Everyone expressed love for Dr. Bozeman! His competence and respectfulness were touted over and over again. A patient who is also a nurse at the hospital commented on how respectful he is of his patients' bodies. He is known to keep unessential areas covered and to insist on gentleness as the body is moved.

But then the discussion began to spiral down into complaining. Patients who had the surgery 6 months to 1 year before talked about being left alone for hours in their hospital beds with no assistance with dressing, walking, going to the bathroom, or getting comfortable in bed. They couldn't even get safety pins to pin their drains to their gowns. Dee quickly noted that the hospital is—as are many—short-staffed when it comes to nurses. I think this is a strong argument for having family or friends with you throughout your stay. Rana and Marlene didn't hesitate to walk with me or help me unplug everything to get up and go to the bathroom. They spent a great deal of time putting the compressors back on my

legs. But they also encouraged my independence and did not stand in my way when I insisted on doing things myself.

The one idea that was expressed over and over again throughout the meeting was: This is serious business and you can die if you don't follow instructions!

Yes, I am glad I attended the support group. It reaffirmed what I already knew to be true—that I am incredibly blessed! I have the proper mindset to accomplish what I need, and I have the right to be proud of myself. The first thing I did when I returned home was to put into effect one of the suggestions given at the meeting. After searching through my cluttered kitchen drawers I found a tape measure and recorded my body measurements: waist, 45 inches; thighs, 31 inches; wrist, 7 inches; breast, 46 inches double Ds; neck, 16 inches; upper arm, 15 inches; hips, 52 inches; and calves, 18 inches.

Back to the Reality of the Everyday

JUNE 11, 2003. As I drove to my office, I caught myself with a mouthful of water that I could not swallow. It scared me when I realized I could not sip because I might gulp instinctively. I stopped at a red light, opened the car door and spit the water out. It was embarrassing. In the past I've always reacted negatively when witnessing others engage in such behavior. Maybe I will be less judgmental in the future. Oh, I hope no one saw that!

In the parking deck I heard my name called. It was Carol Leeman. I waited for her to catch up with me and we walked together. Over my left shoulder was draped a laptop and on the other a canvas bag with papers and food. She quickly grabbed my canvas bag and asked, "Should you be carrying that much stuff after surgery? It isn't pulling on your stitches, is it?"

"I probably shouldn't be carrying this much weight but I don't feel any pulling in my incision or abdomen," I said. I was

glad that she had grabbed the bag because my shoulders were getting tired. As we walked, I talked about my support group experience and how much my surgeon is respected in the community. We talked about the reasons we believe some people don't do what they should and the mind games they must play with themselves. She connected our comments to what we teach in communication about our different selves—the ideal self, the true self, and the perceived self. I enjoy talking with her. She is such a smart lady!

Everyone in our office seems obsessed with weight. In the refrigerator were yogurt, diet soda, Slim-Fast drinks, and a container of strawberries! I was actually happy to see this because it helps keep me in a healthy frame of mind. I put my food in the refrigerator and as I left the kitchen I saw Resa, one of our graduate assistants and one of my former students. She was talking to the secretary, Mary, about her April nuptials. Resa had lost weight! I noticed this immediately. Resa had lost a *lot* of weight! She looked good and I complimented her. No one in the office had noticed or commented on my 20-pound weight loss. I guessed I shouldn't have been surprised. They probably wouldn't really see the difference until I lost 40 pounds or more. Still I suspected that there had been a noticeable weight loss in my face, breasts, thighs, and behind. At least *I* saw it.

Home again, I spoke with a co-worker, Cheryl Spainhour, on the phone. She called to see how I was feeling and to talk about a writing project she was researching. In addition, she said she found the name of the African American student who had written an article on bariatric surgery in one of her journalism classes. I agreed to look up the student's contact information the next day and call her to see if she would give me a copy of the article and discuss it with me.

Marlene called and I told her about the support group meeting. She mentioned that some of her co-workers did not understand why she is considering weight-loss surgery. Even though she

explained our family history to them, they still didn't get it. This discussion with her co-workers took place while they were working a bariatric case in the operating room. Referring to the unconscious patient on the table, a nurse said, "All she needed to do was wire that mouth shut or just push her chair away from the table." Marlene and I agreed individuals who make such comments tend to be thin or have never dieted a day in their lives. Nevertheless, Marlene was concerned about this attitude being prevalent when she got her surgery done there.

Then she brought up the infamous surgeon Dr. Block. Her co-workers were concerned and wanted to make sure that he hadn't been my surgeon. Supposedly, he was doing up to 12 surgeries a day before he was fired by one hospital. The rumor is that he only accepts cash paid up front, provides no aftercare for his patients, and will do the surgery on any outpatient! If true, I am happy that I did not run into this fool. I wonder how long it will take for his actions and greed to catch up with him.

Marlene also mentioned another bariatric case that she had worked that day. A woman who had the surgery in April and lost 50 pounds complained of severe vomiting. The doctor was concerned that her pouch had shrunk or had been damaged in some way. They decided to go in and take a look but did not find anything unusual. The patient was instructed to begin taking a nausea medication that she had stopped. They were able to supply her with some of the drug immediately.

After talking with Cheryl and Marlene, I spoke with my friend Kai. She lives out of state and I wanted to give her an update on my situation. We talked about clothes and the sizes we wear. I mentioned that I had clothes from sizes 12 through 26 in my closet and I was determined not to buy another piece until I was less than a size 12. Kai has been dieting by doing a high-protein, low-carb type of diet like Atkins or the Zone. She had been wearing a size 26 but could get into a size 20 now. I was proud of her. She had thought about having the surgery but didn't have any co-morbidities and her health insurance would not cover it. If I did not have

diabetes, hypertension, high cholesterol, and the other co-morbidities I was diagnosed as having, I would also lose weight the traditional way. But, with these problems, it is very difficult to lose
enough weight to see any true health benefit.

Now for my daily nutritional update: I got in approximately
46 grams of protein by eating ¼ slice whole wheat bread with
reduced-fat American cheese, 2 ounces of Cha Cha Chili protein
soup, 2 ounces of yogurt, 3 ounces of Country Lentil protein soup
with string mozzarella, and a smoothie made with 4 ounces of
milk, 2 ounces of yogurt, and a scoop of protein powder.

THURSDAY, JUNE 12, 2003. During my morning shower I
noticed the remnants of paper tape clinging to my stomach. My
skin is so sensitive and I worry about the damage that may remain.
I avoid putting lotions or anything on my stomach for fear of infection even though it appears that my six incisions are healing nicely.
They aren't ugly. They look like small leaves. Each incision line is
about half an inch long with six small dots around it. The line and
the dots are scabbed over and I'm trying to do everything in my
power to make sure the scabs come off naturally. Of the six incisions, the one that held the drain worries me the most. That area
seems to be more sunken in than the others.

Nutritionally, it was a good day. I got 45 grams of protein in
my food. Once again I had ¼ slice whole wheat with American
cheese, 2 ounces of Cha Cha Chili protein soup with ½ stick of
mozzarella, 2 ounces of yogurt, 3 ounces of Country Lentil soup
with ½ stick of mozzarella cheese, and a smoothie made with 2
ounces of yogurt, 4 ounces of skim milk, and a scoop of protein
powder. Will I soon tire of this menu?

It is amazing how much time we spend on the phone. I think I
talk on the phone more than I do face to face these days. I spoke
with Marlene tonight, and she had shared my first support group
meeting story with a nurse who works primarily with surgeons
who do bariatric surgery. That nurse told her a story about a
bariatric patient who woke up the day after surgery and was so
thirsty that she drank a pitcher of water before anyone could stop

her. Her stomach burst and she ended up with an extended stay in the hospital! "Wasn't someone in the room with her? How could this happen the day after surgery while she was still in the hospital?" I asked. Marlene didn't know.

When I was in the hospital, they didn't even have a pitcher in my room. I don't even remember being thirsty in the hospital. But Marlene reminded me that I slept most of the first day, and when I woke up on the second, the first thing out of my mouth was that I was thirsty. They gave me a 2-ounce cup with 1 ounce of water and a swab. The swab was a little pick sponge on a stick. I was instructed to swab the sponge around the inside of my mouth when thirsty. She was right! I now remembered how nasty and sticky my mouth tasted. I even remembered brushing my teeth over and over again to get that fresh breath feeling and never quite achieving it. How could I forget that?

As I lay thinking about this experience I noted that one of the greatest benefits of this surgery has been my ability to sleep through the night. I used to get up three or four times a night. I would go to sleep by midnight and be awake at 2:30 a.m. watching television and going back and forth to the bathroom until I fell back to sleep around 4:00 or 5:00 a.m. Frequent urination was one of the effects of diabetes, and I was constantly afraid that I might trip and hurt myself as I hurriedly got in and out of the bed. But, no more! Hey, my voice seems stronger and clearer now! Is this my imagination?

FRIDAY, JUNE 13, 2003. A quiet day. I didn't want to do anything or go anywhere. I stayed home and enjoyed watching my soap operas. I didn't write. I didn't read. The only human being I saw was one of the complex workers who came by to check for leaks around my sinks. He found nothing.

I ate an egg made with skim milk and ½ slice of cheese, ¼ slice whole wheat with cheese, 3 ounces of protein soup, 2 ounces of yogurt and something new—a tablespoon of peanut butter! I finished the night with a scoop of protein mixed in 4 ounces of

milk that took me nearly 3 hours to drink. It added up to 48.5 grams of protein. This seemed like a lot of food to me and I felt something was in my mouth at every moment of the day. I didn't like this feeling!

I sneezed for the first time since surgery, and I could feel it reverberating through my upper chest and shoulders. I swear I could feel it force its way through my veins and arteries. It was the strangest sensation I've had—both scary and exhilarating!

SATURDAY, JUNE 14, 2003. I feel good! Lighter. When I look at myself in the mirror, I know that I have lost some of my big butt. Admittedly, I have a long way to go, but my pants seem less stressed at the seams. For the first time I had no trouble putting on my watch. It took less than a second and the watch feels loose on my wrist. I feel so good I decided to go to my office to work. As I drove with a grin on my face and a bottle of water beside me to keep me hydrated, I thought about the enormous folder resting on the passenger's seat that represents my journey through gastric bypass. It contained information on the surgery, diabetes, vaccines, weight-loss programs, and privacy notices. It is a good thing I like to read! Indeed. It has been a good day. I managed to get in 48 grams of protein and found that a smoothie made with 4 ounces of skim milk with 4 ounces of French vanilla yogurt and a scoop of protein powder is tasty. I can't imagine ever going back to drinking Ensure, Boost, or Go-Lean.

SUNDAY, JUNE 15, 2003. One day up, the next one down. I felt incredibly lazy and unmotivated and spent much of the day in bed. I wanted to treat myself to a movie and browse through a bookstore, but it didn't happen. I could not bring myself to get up and *make* a protein shake, let alone drink one; 26 grams of protein was all I managed to consume. Not good. I just didn't feel well, but I wasn't sick enough to call anyone for help. Nauseated, I walked around the house in hope that that would settle my stomach. In between walks, I sat on the floor and did some stretching and arm exercises with 2-pound weights hoping I would feel better. I didn't.

MONDAY, JUNE 16, 2003. I had an appointment with my surgeon. In the waiting room I was irritated because there were two women who just could not stop smacking gum. When the nurse called my name I nearly ran her over to get away from that annoying noise. The nurse weighed me at 224 pounds and showed me to an examination room.

"Didn't I just see you?" Dr. Bozeman teased as he entered the room.

"Yes, I was in a couple of weeks ago to have my drain removed," I reminded him. The nurse entered with another doctor who Dr. Bozeman introduced and said laughingly, "Don't tell him that this surgery cures diabetes. Though it does! Don't tell him that you don't have to take any of those diabetic medicines or anti-hypertension drugs anymore—though you don't!"

Everyone was laughing happily as he wrote the word *off* across a sheet listing the medications I had to take before surgery.

"Do you have any concerns or questions?" Dr. Bozeman asked.

"A week before surgery you insisted that I have a pap smear, but I didn't have the time to do it because of the Memorial Day holiday."

"You must really feel guilty about that, so, yes, go ahead and contact your family doctor and get it done. No, since you did not follow my instructions I think we should have an operation to reverse this surgery next week!" he said jokingly.

I joked, "You can schedule it all you want, but guess who won't be there?"

We all laughed. I was happy! I said that I thought my food choices were too limiting, and Dr. Bozeman told me to trust my nutritionist, that she would not steer me wrong. This was not what I wanted to hear but what I knew I *needed* to hear. He congratulated me for doing well and said I would not need to see him again for 2 months.

As I prepared to check out, the receptionist informed me that I still had $100 due on my account. "Do you want to pay any of it today?" she asked. I gave her the only cash in my wallet, $15.

As far as protein sustenance, it was an excellent day! I got in 62 grams and can really tell the difference in my energy level. My strategy consisted of having two smoothies averaging 28 grams of protein each. I will continue to do this for a while. The trick to feeling good and handling nausea seems to be to drink a protein shake and not eat or drink anything else for at least 45 minutes. I can sip constantly on a clear liquid for an hour, wait 45 minutes or more, then eat or drink again.

DISCUSSION QUESTIONS

1. What is expertise? When information from professionals is inconsistent or contradictory, how do you decide which to follow?

2. What is a support group? Are there any common characteristics we find across effective support groups focusing on health issues?

3. How would you characterize the interaction between the patient and her nutritionist? Which health model(s) do they seem to represent?

4. Is there really any value in keeping a food diary?

5. Are there racial, ethnic, and gender differences in the decision to have major surgery?

6. What do you think about the stories told in the support group? Is the sharing of such information helpful or harmful? Has your perception of weight-loss surgery changed based on these stories? If so, how and why?

7. What are the ethical responsibilities of health professionals? Should health professionals share negative information about other health professionals with their family and friends? Why or why not? Are there any consequences for bad behavior for health professionals, specifically medical doctors?

8. Is humor effective in interactions between doctors and patients? Why or why not?

9. Do things in your work environment support your lifestyle or conflict with it? How might we improve our work environments to be more supportive of healthier lifestyle behaviors?

10. Why do you eat? Does it matter to you what you eat, how, where, and with whom? Explain.

SUGGESTED READINGS

Social Support

Brashers, D. E., Neidig, J. L., & Goldsmith, D. J. (2004). Social support and the management of uncertainty for people living with HIV or AIDS. *Health Communication, 16*(3), 305–331.

Shaw, B. R., Hawkins, R., McTavish, F., & Gustafson, D. H. (2006). Effects of insightful disclosure within computer mediated support groups on women with breast cancer. *Health Communication, 19*(2), 133–142.

Body Image

David, P., Morrison, G., Johnson, M. A., & Ross, F. (2002). Body image, race, and fashion models: Social distance and social identification in third-person effects. *Communication Research, 29*(3), 270–294.

Ferris, J. E. (2003). Parallel discourses and "appropriate" bodies: Media constructions of anorexia and obesity in the cases of Tracey Gold and Carnie Wilson. *Journal of Communication Inquiry 27*(3), 256–273.

Social Identities

Harwood, J. & Sparks, L. (2003). Social identity and health: An intergroup communication approach to cancer. *Health Communication, 15*(2), 145–159.

The Use of Humor

Sala, F., Krupat, E., & Roter, D. (2002). Satisfaction and the use of humor by physicians and patients. *Psychology & Health, 17*(3), 269–281.

Wrench, J. S. & Booth-Butterfield, M. (2003). Increasing patient satisfaction and compliance: An examination of physician humor orientation, compliance-gaining strategies, and perceived credibility. *Communication Quarterly, 51*(4), 482–503.

Health Care Professionalism

Cohen, J. J. (2006). Professionalism in medical education, an American perspective: From evidence to accountability. *Medical Education, 40*(7), 607–617.

7

Week Four Post-Surgery

When a Doctor Leaves a Bad Taste in Your Mouth

TUESDAY, JUNE 17, 2003. I went to the Endocrinology Clinic at NEMC for a visit that was the result of miscommunication and incompetence. I had received a letter scolding me for not keeping a June 2nd appointment even though I had called to reschedule it because I had gotten out of the hospital only two days before. It was my understanding that the appointment was supposed to be scheduled for two weeks post-op. The receptionist thought I didn't have to come in for six weeks, but since I had missed a scheduled appointment, even though it should not have been scheduled at that time, I needed to come in immediately. Although frustrated, I didn't mind because I wanted to meet the other endocrinologists to determine whether or not to stay with this group or have my records sent to Presbyterian Hospital in Charlotte and continue with my former endocrinologist, Dr. Abram Strauss.

I arrived at the office at 8:30 a.m. for my 8:45 a.m. appointment. The receptionist, who was holding my file, asked if this was my first time there. You would think she would take the time to look at the file and determine this. She asked if any of my personal information had changed, then confirmed my birth date, home phone number, and address. I cringed and tried to speak softly as possible but loud enough to not have to repeat what I was saying as others in the waiting area could clearly hear our conversation.

Impatient, I waited for half an hour before a nurse called me back—the longest I had ever waited at this hospital. I was weighed and taken to an examination room where the nurse took my blood pressure (120/72) and my pulse (72) and commented that everything looked fine and that the doctor would be happy. When she left the room, I sat there alone for another half hour.

Dr. Insull Jones entered the room. He did not introduce himself nor did he extend his hand for a handshake as I tried to introduce myself. He immediately sat down and without making eye contact began with, "I see here that you have a nodule on your thyroid and they did a biopsy and didn't find anything. I also see you have diabetes."

I responded, "No, I *had* diabetes. I had gastric bypass surgery and that cured my diabetes."

"Who told you that?" he asked with a slight laugh in his voice.

Caught off guard by his reaction, I said, "My doctor, Dr. Bozeman."

"Isn't he a surgeon? . . . A surgeon cannot make that determination! When did he tell you this?"

"Yesterday."

"Well, that is *our* job. What type of blood tests did he run?"

"I didn't have any blood test yesterday."

As he wrote on a legal pad, he stated, "Well, today you will have blood tests so we can really find out if that is true. You know, you don't know what has changed in your body. In fact, I see here that before the surgery you had very high cholesterol. Did you know that? Do you think that is not the case now, too? Well, one way for us to find out is to have these tests."

He told me to sit on top of the examination table, where he listened to my lungs and stomach, then instructed me to sit once again in the chair. I did as I was told and asked, "How can we confirm that my hypertension has improved or resolved itself?"

The man looked at me as if I was the dumbest person on the face of the earth! With a smirk on his face and laughter in his eyes,

he retorted, "You don't do blood tests to determine hypertension. No, you can't find out about it that way."

He handed the checkout form to me, walked to the door, opened it, and left. No good-bye, it was nice to meet you, good luck, nothing. I was pissed and insulted but took the form to the checkout station and made my co-payment of $28.20. The receptionist scheduled the labs I needed and my next appointment with an endocrinologist on the computer. I told her I did not want to meet with Dr. Jones again and would appreciate seeing another endocrinologist and if that was not possible to just forward my file to Dr. Strauss's office in Charlotte. She assured me that I could see another doctor and stated she was not surprised that I didn't like Dr. Jones. As the other hospital employees in the reception area talked of Dr. Jones's problems with patients, she handed me an appointment slip and instructed me to go downstairs to the laboratory. Things moved relatively fast there; the nurse took three vials of blood and dismissed me.

As I maneuvered through the hallways to find my way out of the hospital, I thought about my interaction with Dr. Jones. I didn't know what to think of him. I know I was disappointed! Unfortunately, I suspect he is the type of doctor who discourages people from ever coming back. I wonder how many people have died . . . how many black folks, because they did not continue with the care they needed because of encounters with asshole doctors like that. Why did he treat me as if I was dirt? As a nobody? As someone unworthy of his time?

I am a highly intelligent, well-educated person, and he made me feel as small as an ant, and I hate him for it! Okay, I dislike him. Good god, my mother is in my head telling me that *hate* is a strong and powerful word. *Are you sure that's what you mean?* No, Ma, you're right, I dislike him a lot . . . No, I dislike his *behavior* a lot.

One thing I do know is that I take it personally when any person of color hurts me or treats others wrong. For some reason I believe *that* behavior reflects on me, on all of us, whether we like

it or not. And, when it comes to taking care of my health, I don't care what color my doctor is, as long as I am treated with respect. If not, he or she will not see me again. I work too hard for my little bit of money to have to deal with a fool then watch him take my hard-earned money!

Hey, give him a break! Maybe he is going through his own stuff right now! After all, doctors are people, too! Right.

Near the entrance to the hospital I ran into a former co-worker, Juanita. We hugged and exclaimed how much we missed one another. Juanita, a white woman, told me about all her health problems and I told her about mine. She looked wonderful, although I was saddened to hear that there were a couple of questionable lumps on her lungs. With her heart disease and recent cauterization, I was concerned. Since she was on her way to an appointment and I was leaving, we hugged and promised to meet sometime for lunch. It was really good to see her! Her hugs reminded me so much of my mother that I was filled simultaneously with overwhelming love and loss. I found myself in tears as I drove home.

My protein count was 42 grams for the day. By 9:00 p.m. I drank only one smoothie and just could not get anything else down. I vowed to try to do better the next day.

Office Talk

WEDNESDAY, JUNE 18, 2003. Another appointment! My week has been busy with appointments. At 8:30 I arrived at my orthodontist's office and approached a smiling assistant who exclaimed, "Oh this will be quick and easy today. We only have to tighten things up!" I knew it would be painful, although I have a high threshold for pain and believe the more the better. The pain in my mouth is confirmation that my teeth are moving into the correct position and my financial investment in braces is worth it. Nevertheless, when I arrived at work and prepared my Cha Cha Chili protein

soup, I struggled to chew the mozzarella stick. It took me an additional twenty minutes to eat every morsel of cheese in the soup to get in 40 grams of protein for the day.

THURSDAY, JUNE 19, 2003. I returned to my office to work. The administrative assistant, Pat, asked how I was feeling and commented that I looked as if I was losing weight. She wanted to know if anything was wrong and if I was mad at her for some reason. Apparently others in the department had approached her with concern for me and she didn't know what to tell them. Our department chair, Rich, had simply told her "it was personal."

I had to tell her something. All the full-time faculty and staff are close, and I knew my secret would soon get out if it hadn't already. When Mary, the secretary, walked into Pat's office, I told them about the gastric bypass surgery. I explained as much as I could about the process and why I felt it was necessary for me to have it—primarily to rid myself of my obesity-related illnesses, especially diabetes, hypertension, and high cholesterol. They were happy for me and proud of me.

We talked about healthy eating and shared information about protein powders. Pat, who was a diet specialist in a former life, uses protein powders. Between the two of us, we convinced Mary to try them. They said my disclosure explained a lot about my behavior in the past few months—distancing myself from them. Both said I should have told them sooner so they could have helped me when I was in the hospital. It would have been easy for them since they lived in the area. Even though I appreciated their expressions of disappointment in not having the opportunity to assist me, I knew *this* was the appropriate time for them to learn my secret. Throughout the year I had become aware of their trials and tribulations and did not want to burden them any further with my own. They support me enough in listening to me as I rant and rave about my classes and students.

When I returned home, I spoke on the phone with Mac, who called to let me know that I had been on her mind. She wanted to know how I was doing. I gave a report of my recent doctor visits

and then we talked about my reasons for having the surgery in the first place. We discussed my mother's sudden illness and slow death and concluded that the long-time use of diabetes medications and the incompetence of a family doctor had led to the demise of a woman who took her health seriously. We were saddened that we were not able to recognize signs or symptoms sooner to help her.

"You are just like your mother. When she made up her mind to do something, she did it," Mac said. "You are the same way. I am proud of you."

The highest compliment you can give me is to compare me favorably to my mother. There is no one I respect or love more.

She asked me about Marlene.

"Marlene and I have had numerous conversations lately in which she indicated that she will be the next to have the surgery," I told Mac. "She is talking more and more about quitting smoking and handling her hypertension. I think she is afraid for her family, especially her husband and daughter."

"Well, maybe your success will inspire them to act soon."

"We can only hope . . ."

". . . and pray."

It is always good to talk with Mac. When she speaks, I hear my mother's voice and see her attitude. Clearly, Mac is one of my guardian angels here on earth. She has dealt with a lot recently— the lupus, kidney dialysis and kidney transplant of her daughter; the death of her best friend; followed six months later by the death of her husband; the convalescence of her oldest son from a heart attack; and the loss of several other friends within months of one another. This woman in her late 70s did everything her doctors asked and even gave a kidney to her daughter—the one thing that I could not do for my own mother and I am in my 40s!

Her faith is amazing and unwavering. Her smile is ever present and illuminating. Mac is a black Mother Teresa without the fame, loved and cherished by many.

Minutes after talking with Mac, the phone rang again. This time it was an aunt who lives in Orlando. We haven't seen or

spoken with each other since my mother's funeral. She bemoaned her life and told me that she had just gotten out of the hospital after experiencing complications from her heart disease and diabetes. She claimed to have lost 40 pounds quickly and was unhappy that none of her eight doctors could explain to her satisfaction why this occurred and swore to rid herself of the "female family doctor who doesn't know what she is doing."

Damn! Another family member experiencing the hell of diabetes and hypertension! I didn't want to hear about it! I didn't want to feel the pain! I didn't want to remember the hell of the past two years! Why was she doing this to me?

I wanted to ask her, *what do you expect me to do? What are you doing about this? What are your children doing to help you?* I didn't. Somehow I convinced myself that it wasn't my business and that I couldn't afford to get emotionally invested in her problems. Then she mentioned that one of her granddaughters is taking care of her. Thank God! When she asked if and when I would be coming for a visit, I told her that I too had recently gotten out of the hospital and wouldn't be traveling long distances for a while. I tried to tell her about the surgery, but she didn't seem interested.

The subject turned to estate matters. My aunt Annie wasn't happy that we sold our mother's house and wanted to know what had happened with the proceeds.

"I paid my mother's debts as required by North Carolina law," I informed her.

"So that is the end of that, huh," she stated in accusatory tone.

"Yes, it is," I replied and hung up.

I have always felt that our conversations are primarily about money, never really about concern for me or my siblings. I have spoken with my aunt in the last year more than I have the entire 40-plus years of my life. If she didn't think she would get something out of our mother's estate, I wouldn't hear from her at all. Now I truly understand the discomfort and sadness my mother exhibited every time she heard from her "sister." Blood doesn't make you family or obligated; it only makes you related.

We took care of our mother when she needed us the most—
the three of us, her children. I know the love and feel the love that
we as siblings have for one another. My sister and her family and
my brother and his family are the only *real* family I have now. My
life is about getting to know them better and getting the love I
need from them. This is what my mother would want. My aunt has
eight children, tens of grandchildren, and who knows how many
great grandchildren. I hope they will do for her what I cannot.

Worn out, I turned the ringer on the phone off and watched
The Oprah Winfrey Show. Oprah announced the re-establishment of
her book club and even more exciting, that Luther Vandross had
been discharged from the hospital to begin physical therapy. I was
happy for him but would really like to know more about his situation. What role did his constant weight gain and loss play in his
stroke? It was reported that his diabetes was under control before
the stroke. Is this true? What will he do differently after he recov-
ers to achieve and maintain good health?

Nauseous, I was only able to get in 41 grams of protein for the
day.

FRIDAY, JUNE 20, 2003. I am focused on nutrition as usual. I
am not happy with my daily protein intake and must find a way to
increase it immediately. I made a smoothie with 4 ounces of skim
milk, 4 ounces of yogurt, and two scoops of protein powder. My
plan was to make one drink containing 52 grams of protein and
savor it throughout the day in three-to-four 2-ounce meals. I
poured the mixture into an empty water bottle to bring it to
work.

In addition, for the first time since my surgery, I snacked on
unsweetened applesauce and made tunafish. Unfortunately, applesauce really doesn't add much nutritional value. It doesn't have any
protein, but it is good. The 3-ounce packet of albacore tuna was
mixed with Miracle Whip, one chopped soft-boiled egg, and cubed
sweet pickles. This dish contained approximately 25 grams of protein. For dinner I ate only one-third of it. Nevertheless, it was a
good day; I managed to get in approximately 60 grams of protein!

SATURDAY, JUNE 21, 2003. I dragged myself out of bed, dressed, took Prevacid and a multivitamin, drank a little Crystal Light, and walked to the complex's clubhouse to get started on my goal to exercise regularly. At the clubhouse I rode the Lifecycle for 20 minutes and then returned to my apartment to do a little housework. I felt good.

For breakfast I tried to eat a scrambled egg although the smell was nauseating. I was determined to eat this high-protein food because I believed it would make my life easier. I have always loved eggs! And, for me, nothing says breakfast like bacon, eggs, and grits!

To make the egg more palatable, I scrambled it with two ounces of American cheese and a drop of skim milk. Then I mixed it with two ounces of grits. I ate as much as I could, felt full, and stopped eating. Nearly one-third of it went into the garbage. At least it tasted better than before—not much better, but better.

I spent most of the day working on campus. Getting out of the house every day gives me an excuse to exercise informally and improves my mood.

Nutritionally, it was an average day with 46 grams of protein consumed.

SUNDAY, JUNE 22, 2003. Dee, my nutritionist, left a message on my voice mail today saying that I could have decaffeinated tea with any non-sugar sweetener. What a relief! I love ice tea! I was getting tired of Crystal Light, water, Jell-O, and Gatorade. I wanted something different! They say "variety is the spice of life," and that cliché has particular relevance for me now. I did absolutely nothing today and got in only 36 grams of protein. Maybe tomorrow I will do better.

MONDAY, JUNE 23, 2003. I could probably commit murder as irritated as I was feeling! It occurred to me that I hadn't had a bowel movement in three or four days. As a result, my plan to stay away from the apartment for most of the day was scrapped, and I found myself on the toilet trying to force a bowel movement. I needed to go to the store and get the Citrucel recommended in my gastric bypass paperwork, but I was afraid to leave the house. If I

had one good movement, then I could go and get the products I needed to avoid this from ever happening again.

Carafate is designed to prevent the development of ulcers within the esophagus and stomach of patients with gastro-esophageal reflux disease (GERD). As I reviewed my post-surgery care paperwork, I read it might cause constipation. Unfortunately, I had already taken my dose of Carafate for the morning, and in anger threw out the nearly empty bottle. Then I tried everything. I poured warm water down my behind. I placed my head between my legs as I sat on the toilet. I pushed my body forward as I sat back against the toilet lid. I pushed, strained, squeezed, and shouted for God's help and even my mother's help, all to no avail. I pushed and squeezed until hemorrhoids developed and all I excreted was blood.

At times I would lie across the bed in an attempt to feel better, although within 10 to 15 minutes I would jump up and head for the bathroom again with the uncontrollable urge to shit. Once I got up, the feeling would subside and I would pace between the bedroom and living room until that became uncomfortable and I found myself once again on the throne. The constant sipping of water as I lay across the bed, walked around the apartment, and as I sat on the toilet did not help. I sat for stretches, even 30 to 45 minutes at a time, until my legs and feet became numb. When I arose, a blacking out sensation would engulf me and I feared dying of dehydration and the inability to shit!

I've never felt as miserable. Before surgery I was as regular as a Swiss clock! Within an hour of eating I would have a bowel movement. Gastric bypass surgery, the drain care, and the drinking of nothing but liquids for days did not compare to the misery of constipation. Now I was beginning to understand how my mother felt as she battled severe constipation on a daily basis throughout her illness. God, I wish I had been more patient and understanding! Is this payback? Laugh, Mom laugh! I deserve it!

My ordeal continued until approximately 5:00 p.m. as *The Oprah Winfrey Show* ended. Sitting on the toilet once again, I decided

I would not push or force something to happen. If it was going to happen, then it would just have to happen on its own. All of a sudden I felt the muscles in my anus contract and push! The contractions were painful and unstoppable. The pushing continued until a string of excrement nearly 10 inches in length and 2 inches in thickness slid out into the water.

What a relief! The joy I felt was equivalent to the joy one feels on the day one commits her life to Jesus. No joke! No shit. No pun intended. Needless to say, I was drained. I was too tired to do anything else that day and prescribed for myself bed rest and a liquid-only diet. Nutritionally, it was an exceptional day with 56 grams of protein and more than 100 ounces of water consumed.

I accept that I will always have to have some form of liquid going into my mouth at all times except for when I am eating or sleeping. A pitcher of water is on the nightstand and if I awaken in the middle of the night, I will take a sip gladly.

Maynard Jackson Jr., the first African-American mayor of Atlanta, died today at the age of 65—the same age my mother was. Jackson, who lived with diabetes and heart disease, collapsed at Reagan National Airport due to cardiac arrest.

Yes, I made the right decision.

DISCUSSION QUESTIONS

1. Are patients consumers with the right to change doctors? Have you ever changed doctors because you were dissatisfied with how you were treated? Explain.

2. What are your privacy rights in the context of health care?

3. Do you care what the gender or race is of your healthcare professionals? Why or why not? What does the academic literature tell us about the impact of racial and gender similarities and differences between doctors and patients on patient care and satisfaction?

SUGGESTED READINGS

Auslander, W. F., Thompson, S. J., Dreitzer, D., & Santiago, J. V. (1997). Mothers' satisfaction with medical care: Perceptions of racism, family stress, and medical outcomes in children with diabetes. *Health and Social Work, 22*, 190–199.

Beck, C., Ragan, S. L., & du Pré, A. (1997). *Partnership for health: Building relationships between women and health caregivers.* Mahwah, NJ: Lawrence Erlbaum Associates.

Cooper, L. A., Roter, D. L., Johnson, R. L., Ford, D. E., Steinwachs, D. M., & Powe, N. R. (2003). Patient-centered communication, ratings of care, and concordance of patient and physician race. *Annals of Internal Medicine, 139*(2), 907–915.

Dixon, L. D. (2004). A case study of an intercultural health care visit: An African American woman and her White male physician. *Women and Language, 27*(1), 45–52.

Gabbard-Alley, A. S. (1995). Health communication and gender: A review and critique. *Health Communication, 7*, 35–54.

Gabbard-Alley, A. S. (2000). Explaining illness: An examination of message strategies and gender. In B. B. Whaley (Ed.), *Explaining illness* (pp. 147–170). Mahwah, NJ: Lawrence Erlbaum Associates.

Johnson, R. L., Saha, S., Arbelaez, J. J., Beach, M. C., & Cooper, L. A. (2004). Racial and ethnic differences in patient perceptions of bias and cultural competence in health care. *Journal of General Internal Medicine, 19*, 101–110.

Roter, D. L., Stewart, M., Putnam, S. M., Lipkin, M. Jr., Stiles, W., & Inui, T. S. (1997). Communication patterns of primary care physicians. *Journal of the American Medical Association, 277*, 350–357.

White, R. A. (2004). Is empowerment the answer? Current theory and research on development communication. *The International Journal for Communication Studies, 66*(1), 7–24.

8

Weeks Five and Six Post-Surgery

TUESDAY, JUNE 24, 2003. I got up and prepared to go to Fayette-ville to take care of some estate business. Nearly a year and a half had passed since my mother's death and I was still settling the estate. I hoped this will be my last meeting with the attorney as we completed the paperwork for the final accounting.

Fayetteville is a three-hour drive from Charlotte and this would be my first long-distance trip alone since the surgery. I got up at 5:45 a.m. and packed the water and protein drink I would need. I was on the road by 7:00 a.m. and arrived for my 10:00 a.m. appointment with the estate attorney at 9:45 a.m. During our meeting I drank most of the protein drink I had prepared, which seemed like a good thing until I realized I had gas. By the time I got to my brother's home, all I could do was knock on the door, push my way in past him, and head for the bathroom. Sweating and tired, I just wanted to rid my body of the gas so my bloated stomach could rest! Tim, concerned, asked if I was alright as he waited outside of the bathroom. I mumbled that I was okay then spent nearly 15 minutes stinking up his bathroom.

It was a good visit with Tim and Virginia. They were support-ive of my decision to have weight-loss surgery, expressed admira-tion for the courage I displayed in having it done in secrecy, and complimented my weight loss and strength to follow through with all of the post-operative rules. As we spoke, gas slowly progressed through my esophagus and out my mouth, bubble upon bubble. We laughed, teased, and debated who spent the most time in the bathroom and whose shit stunk the worst. I felt better.

At 2:00 p.m. I drove back to Charlotte. When I arrived, I called Marlene to let her know I was back, and she convinced me to go to the store immediately to stock up on anti-gas and anti-constipation products. I went to the local grocery store and purchased Citrucel, a B-complex vitamin, the new smooth-dissolve variety of Tums with calcium, and yogurt. Home once again, I mixed a teaspoon of the Citrucel with two ounces of yogurt and ate it. If I have to use Citrucel for the rest of my life, so be it! No more constipation! . . . One can only hope! At the end of the day, I had consumed 40 grams of protein.

WEDNESDAY, JUNE 25, 2003. I got up early and took my Prevacid, multivitamin, and tried to eat as much as possible of my scrambled egg with cheese. With breakfast I took two Tums and tried to swallow the B-complex vitamin, but it had a strong unpleasant smell and my throat rejected it. I gave up and decided I would try again at dinner. My dislike for the size and smell of the capsule prompted me to call Dee to ask if she would recommend a smaller B-complex vitamin. She informed me that I could find a brand (B-Complex 113-188) at the pharmacy in the Medical Arts Building of NEMC, or the Sundowne brand at Lowe's with tablets the size of an aspirin. These would be good options if for some reason I still could not swallow the capsules I had already purchased.

For dinner I ate tunafish with egg, took two Tums, and attempted to take the B-complex vitamin. Once again my throat rejected it and I knew that I would have to purchase a different brand. To handle my constipation, I had Citrucel mixed with applesauce and Crystal Light, twice. My total number of grams of protein for the day was 49.

I found that I have been able to get in more protein through soups and eggs without an overwhelming feeling of fullness lately (June 26, 48 grams, June 27, 46 grams). Taking the Tums has made the gaseous feelings subside tremendously, although my bowel movements remain irregular. Even though I've increased my consumption of liquids, I am still not getting enough water into my system.

Marlene visited during this time, and I appreciated her consideration around meals. We would pick her up something from one of her favorite restaurants and bring it home. I would eat according to my diet protocol and she would eat her meal. We sat in a way that we could comfortably talk and didn't subject me to seeing foods I once ate and in which I could no longer indulge. She avoided putting foods in the refrigerator that she knew I couldn't have, and she didn't leave snack foods on the counter. In some ways being single is an advantage, especially after having weight-loss surgery. It would be incredibly difficult to deal with meals if I had a husband and children. Watching others eat doesn't necessarily bother me. It doesn't make me long for certain foods I know I shouldn't have. For now, anyway, the smell of fatty or sugar-filled foods makes me nauseated.

I think a lot about meat. I've always been the stereotypical meat and potatoes–type person and wouldn't mind having a piece of fried fish! Of course, I've been advised to avoid fried foods, although I find it difficult to wrap my mind around cooking baked, broiled, or stewed fish. I don't know how. Plus, in my mind, the taste of baked, broiled, and stewed fish could never match that of fried fish! My sister-in-law, Virginia, who is adept at cooking fish, has offered to teach me, although we don't see each other enough to make it worth my while. And I must admit that I really do not want to invest the time in learning, especially since I like and can cook other meats such as chicken in a variety of ways.

Chicken! I get to eat chicken and turkey next week! I have been dreaming about baking a chicken thigh and coating it with barbecue sauce. It is heaven! I don't care if it takes me three meals to eat one thigh. No, it is not about being hungry. It is about that feeling of satisfaction you get when you have finished a meal that just makes you feel loved. I miss the contrast of vegetables and fruit, the clash of colors and texture that one gets from a variety of foods. Six weeks post-op can't come soon enough. Then I can have a little meat, vegetable, and fruit in one meal!

My protein intake for Saturday and Sunday, June 28 and 29, was good at 50 grams and 53 grams. The addition of tuna with egg and peanut butter boosts the protein gram count considerably. My goal is to become less dependent on protein powder and eat what passes as more "normal" meals.

One benefit of having this surgery is the definite health-related outcomes from being forced to avoid sugars and fats. My skin is glowing, soft, and seems less dry than previous summers. My hair needs less moisturizer and my knees have not squeaked or been in pain since the surgery. Of course, this may be the result of daily stretches and multivitamins, too.

MONDAY, JUNE 30, 2003. I went shopping for the chicken I can add to my diet beginning tomorrow. The local grocery store has a wide selection of fresh and prepackaged fish with directions on how to cook it. I bought fresh cod that could be prepared with Italian dressing and some chicken thighs. Nutritional charts hung above the meats, and I noted a 4-ounce chicken thigh has 23 grams of protein. It occurred to me that if I eat two pieces of chicken a day, I will get in my required amount of daily protein.

The day was noneventful with 49 grams of protein consumed.

TUESDAY, JULY 1, 2003. I baked four chicken thighs and covered them with barbecue sauce. I was excited to have something different and ate 2 ounces of chicken at breakfast, lunch, dinner, and as snacks. Solid food is much more satisfying, and I had no problem reaching my nutritional goal of 48 grams of protein.

On the bookshelf of my home office, I found *The Complete Book of Food Counts*, which lists nutritional information such as protein, sodium, carbohydrate, and calories for many foods. Even the nutritional values of some foods at popular fast food restaurants were listed. I placed the book on the dinning room table for easy reference as I add new foods to my diet.

It is the first Tuesday of the month, the day the support group meets. I made the 20-minute drive to Concord in the pouring rain and went straight to the pharmacy to get the B-complex vitamin Dee recommended. The pharmacy, located at the entrance to the hospital, was small and crowded with a long line of people at the register. I looked on the shelves where the vitamins were located but did not see any B-complex vitamins, then stood in line for nearly 15 minutes hoping that the cashier would be able to assist me. The line did not move and I decided to try again later.

I walked downstairs toward the classroom where we met previously. Around the theater area were displays on the history of the medical center. The historical display began in the 1930s and concluded in the 1980s. One display noted the hospital had served "Negroes" in the 1930s because there were no other medical facilities for them at the time. The "Negro" community provided the furniture and equipment for the rooms on the "Negro ward," and "Negro" nurses were hired to take care of the "Negro" patients. In addition, a picture of the longest working "Negro" nurse, who was also thought to be the oldest living person in North Carolina at the time, hung on the wall. She was dressed in her Sunday best and sitting in a chair. She was beautiful! The plaque beneath her photo indicted she worked until she was 107 and died at the age of 108.

I was proud that she had survived and worked many years, although another part of me felt sad that she may have had to work that long. I thought about how things change but still manage to stay the same. Because of her efforts and those of many unnamed and unrecognized others, I will never have to experience a "Negro" ward. I have the status and privilege to be just another well-insured individual getting the best medical science has to offer.

Nevertheless, as I looked at the display of nurses and doctors from the 1950s through the 1980s, I did not see another person of color.

It was five minutes until the meeting was scheduled to begin, although no one else had arrived. Then a woman carrying bottled water descended the stairs and looked into each of the three empty classrooms. She sat and waited outside of classroom #3. I introduced myself and we spent the next 20 to 25 minutes talking as we waited for the others to show up.

Dana had had her surgery three days after mine and commented that her pouch "was smaller than it was supposed to be." She never stated how she knew this or why it was the case, and I didn't ask.

"How much have you lost?" she asked.

"Oh, I'm not sure. I haven't been weighed in nearly two weeks. I only get weighed at the doctor's office, but my last calculated loss was 25 pounds."

"I can't believe you don't know how much you've lost," she exclaimed. "I weigh myself every day! I have to weigh myself every day! Do you know it took me a month to lose 26 pounds? I thought I would have lost a whole lot more by now. I'm really disappointed, but I try to tell myself that there is no other way I could lose as much as I have in such a short time."

She said she spoke with our surgeon regularly about nutrition, which surprised me. She didn't want to confer with our nutritionist who she saw as less of an expert. It disturbed me that she would bother a busy surgeon with questions about food when we have an excellent nutritionist. I didn't feel confident the surgeon could answer my questions concerning diet.

In addition, she confessed she did not like soft foods and started eating solid foods immediately upon leaving the hospital. She also did not drink liquids exclusively for the two weeks post-surgery as recommended. Nevertheless, she was having difficulty getting in enough protein and primarily ate high-protein nutrition bars. This resulted in severe constipation problems that she did not know how to solve. I suggested Dee's advice to twice daily drink one teaspoon of Citrucel mixed with 2 to 3 ounces of liquid or yogurt. She thought one tablespoon of Citrucel had to be diluted in 8 ounces of water before consumption. If so, we would never get relief! It felt good to share advice and experiences. We both commented on how comforting it was to talk with someone else who had the surgery around the same time. At around 6:30 it occurred to us that the meeting wasn't taking place and we walked to the parking lot together, said our good-byes, and promised to see each other at the next meeting.

Later that evening, I had an exciting phone conversation with my sister. Good news! She completed all of the preliminary paperwork and would meet with her bariatric surgeon for the first time the next day.

WEDNESDAY, JULY 2, 2003. On the phone, Amy, the assistant from the nutritionist's office, told me the support group would meet the following Tuesday. A cosmetic surgeon would join us as our guest speaker. She apologized for the mix-up and got my e-mail address to make sure I would get messages about future events and changes.

Throughout the day, I ate meat. For both breakfast and lunch, I had chicken, which seems to fill me up comfortably and gives me a sense of satisfaction. I prepared Alaskan cod with Italian dressing and baked it to have for dinner. I did not like it and so I didn't eat it. The meat was tough and the smell was nauseating! Disappointed and frustrated, I went to the grocery store and purchased lightly breaded fish fillets from the frozen foods section and oven-roasted turkey from the deli. Mrs. Paul's lightly battered flounder fillets are approximately 2.5 ounces with low fat, sugar, and carbohydrate content and 10 grams of protein per fillet. These fillets were good and I was able to get in 39 grams of protein for the day.

Marlene called after her consultation at the bariatric surgeon's office. They gave her more paperwork to fill out and instructed her to get a referral to see a psychologist from her family doctor. She is required to go to informational meetings conducted by the surgeon and have a variety of medical tests that would not be completed until the end of August. Apparently her actions have inspired her husband, who, to our surprise, turned up at the surgeon's office for a consultation. I wonder if his sudden interest in the surgery is out of concern for his health or a need to compete with his wife. Marlene attempted to convince Reggie for months that the surgery would improve his knees and overall health, and he insisted it was not for him. Regardless of his reasons for seriously considering the surgery, I am proud that my sister, who has spent her life taking care of others, is finally putting herself first.

THURSDAY, JULY 3, 2003. The day began miserably. I wanted to have a bowel movement before my appointment, but it didn't happen. My problem with constipation continues. Nevertheless, I was anxious to see Dr. May Land, my family doctor, and hear the results of my blood tests taken three weeks ago. I want to know if my glucose is under control, what my cholesterol levels are, and if I will be required to go back on any of the medications I took before surgery. I did not want to have a pap smear, although I knew I would if she insisted; I had put it off too many times. The plan was to avoid being talked into having a full-blown physical. In my mind I had had one every month for nearly six months. No one would take my blood today!

At the doctor's office, a nurse weighed me. I lost only one pound in two weeks! Disappointed and on the verge of crying, I thought my failure to lose more had to be a result of the constipation. I believe if I can shit, I would lose 2 to 3 more pounds! The nurse took my blood pressure, which was good at 118/84, and I undressed for the pap smear and breast examination. Dr. Land performed both tests and then looked in the file for the report of my recent blood tests from my endocrinologist. Unfortunately, the endocrinologist, Insull Jones, had not sent the results—only a letter stating he had taken blood tests and would send them when available. Dr. Land assured me that she would contact me immediately with the results so we could determine whether I needed to take any medications. She congratulated me on my weight loss and admitted she was surprised at how well I looked after having surgery recently. In addition, she inquired if I was following the diet and exercising as instructed, and reminded me to schedule my yearly mammogram for sometime in September. My co-payment for this office visit was $15.

From home I called the endocrinologist and left a message that I wanted my test results, then called the nutritionist to see what I could do about my continued constipation. I reminded her that I was taking one teaspoon of Citrucel in 2 to 3 ounces of liquid twice a day. Dee suggested I try 30 cc's of Milk of Magnesia once or twice a day and one Colace capsule. Our conversation turned to weight loss when I expressed disappointment at losing only one pound in two weeks. She told me not to get excited or be concerned, that this was normal. She said that individuals go through periods of two to three weeks without any weight loss and that I would more than likely lose more weight by our next appointment. At that time we would reassess whether or not things were going as they should. This conversation did comfort me.

After speaking with Dee, I called my sister. Marlene reiterated that the body has to adjust and readjust to weight loss and it would be unhealthy to lose weight each week at the rate of my first two weeks. Later that afternoon, my call to the endocrinologist was returned by the physician assistant. My blood tests were normal, including the glucose, cholesterol, and lipids, even though my calcium was a little high. "It is nothing to be concerned about. You're going to live!" she stated with a laugh.

Now I guess I can claim that my diabetes and hypertension are cured. Can't I?

Sixty-three grams of protein were consumed today.

FRIDAY, JULY 4, and our nation is celebrating its independence. Not me. I do not want to be tempted by holiday foods and damage my stomach. Throughout the day I ate flounder and chicken to satisfy my need for taste and nutrition. In addition, I had a cruel reminder of why it is essential to take care of myself. Barry White, the soulful baritone of love songs, died today of kidney failure. The 58-year-old lived with chronic high-blood pressure then had a stroke while waiting for a kidney transplant. Fifty-eight years old! So young!

Throughout the weekend I concentrated on taking Citrucel twice daily. I even had a burst of energy on Saturday and went to my office to decorate a board announcing a new track for the major in Communication Studies. Plus, my nutritional intake was exceptional with an average of 53 grams of protein. With the inclusion of meat in my diet I find it easier to get in the required protein, and I still have at least one smoothie a day for convenience. Nonetheless, I am a little depressed. I keep looking at myself in the mirror and I don't see enough changes in my body. I feel and look fat. The bathroom scale has become my enemy.

DISCUSSION QUESTIONS

1. What is the racial and gender history of your favorite hospital? How does knowledge of this history make you feel?

2. Why do we tease each other about "having gas" and other bodily functions?

3. How do your interactions with and around food affect those around you?

4. Does the size of one's household shape one's attitudes toward food? How are those values or beliefs verbalized?

5. How are health professionals such as nutritionists viewed in comparison with medical doctors such as surgeons? To what does the term "expertise" refer, and is expertise transferable? Are some health professionals viewed as less knowledgeable because their profession is dominated by a specific gender? Explain.

6. Do you experience uncertainty when you meet a stranger for the first time? How is your uncertainty verbalized? Do we tell strangers things we wouldn't tell our closest friends? Why or why not?

THEORIES TO FACILITATE DISCUSSION WITH SUGGESTED READINGS

Co-Cultural Theory argues the ideas of silencing, giving voice, and marginalization are useful in understanding the lived experiences of a variety of cultural groups. The theorist, Mark Orbe, has identified several co-cultural communication practices utilized by members of various co-cultures when encountering members of the dominant culture.

Orbe, M. P. (1998). *Constructing co-cultural theory: An explication of culture, power, and communication.* Thousand Oaks, CA: Sage.

Social Exchange Theory suggests we think of our relationships in economic terms and keep a count of the costs and rewards of maintaining a relationship. The theory predicts that the value (positive or negative) we place on a relationship influences whether we will continue or end that relationship. For more information read:

Monge, P. R., & Contractor, N. (2003). *Theories of communication networks.* Oxford: University Press.

Raschick, M., & Ingersoll-Dayton, B. (2004). The costs and rewards of caregiving among aging spouses and adult children. *Family Relations, 53,* 317–325.

Standpoint Theory suggests our experiences, knowledge, and communication behaviors are shaped by the social and cultural groups to which we belong. These groups provide us with a perspective or way of making sense of our everyday lived experiences. For more information read:

Bell, K. E., Orbe, M. P., Drummond, D. K., & Camara, S. K. (2000). Accepting the challenge of centralizing without essentializing: Black feminist thought and African American women's communicative experiences. *Women's Studies in Communication, 23,* 41–62.

Hartsock, N. (1998). *The feminist standpoint revisited and other essays.* Boulder, CO: Westview Press.

Uncertainty Reduction Theory explains what happens when strangers meet and converse with one another for the first time. It suggests strangers are primarily concerned with reducing any uncertainty they feel about one another while simultaneously increasing their ability to predict what will happen next in the encounter. For more information read:

Berger, C. R., & Calabrese, R. J. (1975). Some explorations in initial interaction and beyond: Toward a developmental theory of interpersonal communication. *Human Communication Research, 1,* 99–112.

Gudykunst, W. B., & Hammer, M. R. (1987). The influences of ethnicity, gender, and dyadic composition on uncertainty reduction in initial interactions. *Journal of Black Studies, 18,* 191–214.

In addition, these general communication texts have excellent chapters or summaries of the aforementioned theories.

Miller, K. (2005). *Communication theories: Perspectives, processes, and contexts* (2nd ed.). New York: McGraw-Hill.

West, R. & Turner, L. H. (2007). *Introducing communication theory: Analysis and application* (3rd ed.). New York: McGraw-Hill.

9

Weeks Seven, Eight, and Nine Post-Surgery

JULY 8, 2003. I signed in at 6:00 p.m. and joined the 45 to 50 individuals in attendance for the support group. For the first time there were other African Americans present—three in all including me! One had the operation more than a year ago and the other was preparing to have the surgery. Lisa, who had the surgery, looked fantastic. She wore a shape-revealing, sleeveless, above-the-knee jean dress and a broad white-toothed smile. You could see the smoothness of her skin and the muscles in her arms. She was the smallest person in the room, and everyone was looking at her with envy. Or was it hope? I felt both.

Dee began the meeting by handing out a sheet entitled "Steps to Success with Bariatric Surgery." It listed seven habits that patients need to develop to maintain weight loss after surgery, including avoiding carbonated beverages and caffeine, choosing healthy foods to eat, having caring people around for support, exercising at least four times a week for at least 40 minutes, taking vitamins, and getting enough sleep. The seventh habit suggested one hold oneself personally responsible for one's achievements. In addition, the sheet reminded us that the surgery was only a tool—success depended on long-term lifestyle changes, and making such lifestyle changes would be hard work but the best gift we would ever give ourselves.

The guest speaker was Dr. Dave Kidron, a plastic surgeon. He said that plastic surgery after weight loss is designed to reduce "significant redundant skin." Such surgery is for cosmetic reasons with no health benefit and therefore not covered by health insurance. Redundant skin has lost its elasticity and cannot "bounce back," regardless of the type of exercise one does, including weight lifting. "It is a physical impossibility to mend stretch marks," he said. Hanging skin is not unhealthy, but it isn't aesthetically pleasing. Typical problem areas for many gastric bypass patients include the breasts, neck, abdomen, underarms, thighs, and face.

Dr. Kidron recommended that those considering plastic surgery be patient and "use a staged approach" to improve problem areas. One should not try to get everything done in one day because it would cause too much stress on the body. First, he recommended, achieve your goal weight and maintain stability for a year. Most gastric bypass surgery patients have been at a stable weight for at least a year before plastic surgery although a few have had plastic surgery after only six months of stability.

He talked about the types of surgeries he did *not* like to perform. Surgery on the underside of the upper arm area was his least favorite because it usually results in a long ugly scar that patients feel they must cover with short or long sleeves. New techniques are being developed to address this issue. One involves placing the scar under the underarm, although this is considered riskier because the scar is situated near key blood vessels.

In addition, Dr. Kidron talked about the risks of cosmetic surgery and other issues one should seriously consider before proceeding. The development of blood clots and resulting death is always possible. If a patient is a smoker, there is a greater probability of blood vessels constricting during surgery, resulting in stroke, heart attack, or death. *Most* routine cosmetic surgery is done on an outpatient basis, but gastric bypass patients are hospitalized, a decision that is made case-by-case, based on the health status of the patient. Hospitalization adds considerably to the cost of plastic surgery. In addition, patients must plan for a minimum of three weeks recovery time.

Some other problems experienced by plastic surgery patients include keloids, rashes, and moles. Keloids, severe scaring that is raised on the skin and rarely diminishes in appearance, are common in African Americans although found in all groups. It is particularly a problem for individuals who have a family history of keloids occurring around ear piercing. Dr. Kidron continued with advice on dealing with rashes and irritated moles in the breast and thigh areas as one loses weight. He suggested keeping the areas as dry as possible and going without a bra. If one didn't want to go without a bra, one could put a soft cloth between the band of the bra and the irritated area to prevent rubbing. Individuals receiving plastic surgery on the abdomen or thighs would need to be pre-pared to wear a girdle or bodysuit for four weeks or more. A lower body lift involving the thighs, buttocks, and abdomen is the most extensive and dangerous plastic surgery one can have, requiring the longest recuperation time.

Many of the attendees wanted information about breast sur-gery. Dr. Kidron began by explaining the difference between a breast lift and a breast reduction. Breast reductions, unlike breast lifts, provide a health benefit for the patient and are covered by health insurance. They are rarer than many people realize because a physician must make the argument that 300 grams or more of material will need to be removed to improve back and neck pain. A breast lift is automatic with a breast reduction. Most weight-loss patients have lost substantial breast material and do not need more taken out. What they want or need is a lift to improve sagging. Over and over again Dr. Kidron reiterated that even if one has a lift "gravity will never give up." He said, "Skin always relaxes and even-tually the breast will sag again."

Dr. Kidron is one of approximately 5,000 plastic surgeons in the United States. He performs between 40 and 50 breast reduc-tions and lifts a year in the operating suites of his own clinic. He does liposuction and, for safety reasons, will not remove more than 5 liters at a time. Dr. Kidron even corrects inverted nipples! If you did not have one as a child or young adult and then develop one, it is indicative of breast cancer.

When the meeting ended, many of the attendees remained, mingling and talking with each other. Friends got together and took pictures commemorating their weight loss. Individuals introduced themselves to the new potential patients and encouraged them to proceed with the surgery. Others discussed their perceptions of the various doctors they encountered.

I learned a lot today! It turns out that attending support groups is not a waste of my time. Nevertheless, I cannot see myself having or even *considering* having plastic surgery in the future. Although, who knows, if I can't get this tummy flat, I might consider a tuck!

FRIDAY, JULY 11, 2003. I went to Dee's for our one-on-one monthly nutrition consultation. She asked me to get on the scale, took my weight, and recorded the 222 pounds in her notebook. We were both concerned that I had lost only six pounds in four weeks. She asked how much water I drank and how much exercise I did each day. I told her that I drank at the most 32 ounces of water and walked 15 to 20 minutes a day. She instructed me to increase my walks by 10 minutes and my water intake to 48 ounces a day.

Dee measured my blood pressure at 102/70 and reviewed the results of my latest blood tests with me. My lipids, cholesterol, and blood sugars were all in healthy ranges. She even commented that my cholesterol was better than hers at 154. Again, however, my calcium was higher than normal. Dee admitted she did not know what, if anything, this indicated, but would contact my endocrinologist to find out. We spent the rest of our time together discussing the points on the handout she provided me. I could now add one tablespoon of a vegetable or fruit to my meals and try to build up to two tablespoons. An entire meal at this point could be 3 ounces. The sheet laid out various combinations

of food one might start off with, such as 2 ounces of fi[
tablespoon of green beans or steamed broccoli. I v[
taste-test any new food I incorporated into my diet to see if it
agreed with me and to wait a while before trying again any food
that didn't. Apparently, it is not uncommon for one's taste in food
to change after gastric bypass surgery.

Dee reiterated the need to continue to get in 45 to 65 grams
of protein per day, to eat two meals and three snacks, and to wait
45 minutes after eating before drinking any fluids. Otherwise, liquids were to be consumed continuously throughout the day. I
could eat a variety of high-protein bars. Any high-protein bar I ate
had to be less than 250 calories with less than 13 grams of sugar,
low in fat, and have a minimum of 2 grams of fiber. I was reminded
to carefully measure my food, chew thoroughly, eat slowly, and
exercise continuously. Finally, Dee made it clear that the incorporation of starches such as potatoes and rice into my diet was not an
option at this time.

When I left the consultation I went grocery shopping. I was
happy about my test results but dismayed at my weight loss and
admitted to myself that I wasn't exercising enough. I vowed to
become more physically active. Shopping for food may be fun
although expensive, especially when shopping for good quality
meats. Trying to find protein bars that fit the limitations of my diet
was an even bigger challenge. Many protein bars cost over $2.00
each and contain 25 grams or more of sugar. I purchased a variety
of bars fitting my nutritional requirements to taste-test.

At home I phoned the personal trainer who had been assigned
to me to schedule a fitness consultation. Unfortunately, he would
not be able to meet with me for a couple of weeks. He was taking
some time off to enjoy and assist in the birth of his baby. Disappointed, I drove to the YMCA across from my apartment complex
and got information about swimming lessons. Again, my timing
was off. It was too late to sign up for classes and there was a waiting list for private lessons. I had my name added to the list. I was

beginning to feel there was this invisible force trying to prevent me from following through with my vow to make exercise a serious part of my life. But I wouldn't let it stop me!

Throughout the next few days, from Tuesday through Monday (July 8–14), I averaged 54 grams of protein. I noticed that my water intake increased because my output in the mornings and before bedtime seemed to be much more than before. In addition, I added red meat to my diet, which made me feel I was getting the type of variety I needed to thrive. I ate meats, protein bars, fruits, and vegetables, and drank 48 ounces of bottled water every day.

SATURDAY, JULY 12, 2003. I started keeping an exercise record. My apartment complex has a relatively sophisticated work-out room with treadmills, bikes, weight machines, mats, and free weights and I made use of it for four days in a row. I challenged myself to go full force on the treadmill and bike, and I averaged 37 minutes per workout. Before, during and after, I drank consider-able amounts of water to remain hydrated, and the amount of sweat that drenched my clothes became my yardstick for success. When I left the gym, I was tired, but I felt good!

JULY 15–JULY 21, 2003. I haven't had a protein shake in two weeks! Fish, pork chops, hamburger, chicken, and a variety of fruits and vegetables, including peaches, pineapples, pears, spinach, green beans, and brussel sprouts have become the staples of my diet. I continue to take a multivitamin, calcium, and Pre-vacid on a daily basis; average 54 grams of protein and 35 minutes of aerobic exercise per day on the treadmill or bike. One major benefit of regular exercise is regular bowel movements. Actually, it is probably the combination of eating solid foods and exercising that is working. Since I've been working out regularly, I've had a bowel movement every morning. I have decided to discontinue the Colace and take Citrucel only once a day to see what happens.

I feel lighter and my legs look firmer. Before surgery, I would become bloated and my sweat tasted salty when exercising. Now my sweat tastes like the bottled water I drink all day. I needed to know if I am losing weight, so I broke down and purchased a high-quality scale. When I got the scale home, I weighed myself and discovered I had lost six pounds in the past week! I was excited but immediately began to doubt the accuracy of the scale and found myself weighing myself over and over again to see if the number changed. Obsessed with weighing myself every hour and concerned by this behavior, I talked myself into weighing once every three days. My obsession turned to assessing the accuracy of the scale. I called Dee to set up an appointment to weigh myself so I could compare the scales.

To distract myself from the scale, I watched television. On one program, either *Inside Edition* or *Entertainment Tonight,* they announced Randy Jackson, one of the stars from the reality show, *American Idol*, had gastric bypass surgery last week. Supposedly he was unhappy with contestants' comments about his weight. They did not mention any co-morbidity that may have played a role in his decision to have the surgery. I wonder . . .

JULY 22–JULY 28, 2003. Another week dedicated to eating as prescribed and exercising. I continued to take my multivitamin, calcium, and Prevacid, while my daily protein intake averaged 55 grams and I exercised 45 minutes per day on the treadmill or bike. The more I exercise, the more I want to. For example, on Monday morning I had an 8:00 a.m. appointment with my orthodontist. I got up too late to get in a 40 to 50 minute workout. As a result, the entire time I was at the orthodontist I thought about the energizing effects of exercising first thing in the morning. The minute I returned home, I exercised. Therefore, I will try to work out at least five days a week. Seven days a week seems impossible. I am convinced that my success in losing weight will be based on exercising consistently. Two weeks ago I was concerned about my weight leveling off. Although, since then I have exercised regularly and lost another 11 pounds!

On July 25, I celebrated my 44th birthday with Marlene, her family and church members in the basement of their African

Methodist Episcopal church. Food was in abundance and included potato salad, fried chicken, Buffalo wings, sausage, pimento dip with chips, cakes, pies, and homemade lemonade. I knew there wouldn't be anything there that I could eat and came prepared with my own foods. Many of the guests did not know I had had weight-loss surgery and those who did know did not harass or pressure me to eat the foods they prepared. I was proud of myself because I loved every food displayed but remained unfazed. Plus, I was complimented often on my weight loss.

Later that night, close to midnight, my niece and nephew convinced their father to go out and pick them up some hamburgers and French fries from Wendy's. I was asked if I wanted anything and responded "no." My niece commented, "I am not used to you not eating with us." At any other time this statement might have saddened me, but it didn't this time. I want my niece to see and understand that I have made a serious lifestyle change and that commitment to better health entails sacrifice. The best way to make my point is to set the example for her because I believe her life, too, is threatened by obesity.

AUGUST 2003. The weeks are beginning to run together as my new eating and exercise behaviors become routine. I continue taking multivitamins, B-12, Prevacid, Tums for calcium and to control gas, and Citrucel to prevent constipation, and I average 55 grams of protein per day. I exercise for five days out of seven for 50 minutes, and my meals consist of 2 ounces of protein in the form of chicken or lean red meat. To make the Citrucel more palatable, I have learned to mix one teaspoon in 2 ounces of yogurt and then follow that with 2 ounces of milk 15 minutes later. I still find it difficult to eat three meals and two snacks each day, especially when I try to complete all my meals by 7:00 p.m. To eat all my meals and get in a minimum of 48 ounces of water, I have to eat breakfast as early as 7:00 a.m. and continue eating and drinking until 9:00 p.m. I am rarely hungry and have to force myself to eat.

When I met with my physical trainer for the first time, the exercise room was much smaller than I expected. It had four television sets, exercise bikes, treadmills, and elliptical, step, and weight machines arranged in a circle around a small track. The track was so small that it would take 23 trips around it to make a mile! I was disappointed to discover the gym did not have a pool; I wanted to learn how to swim and take a water aerobics class. Everyone in the room was white and old. The room smelled like old people. I did not feel comfortable or particularly welcomed. My young, white male trainer explained that because it was a Friday afternoon, the gym would be relatively empty. He was right. I saw eight people the entire time I was there. Mr. Miller spent much of his time sharing the pictures of his newborn with the patrons and trying to sell me a membership to the gym. Without an immediate commitment to purchase a membership, I was informed I would be entitled to only an eight-minute walking test and instruction on how to use the free medium-strength Dyna-Band® he would provide me.

Mr. Miller was obligated to explain the results to me of my Personal Wellness Profile based on a survey I completed when I first met with my nutritionist. The profile was an overview of my exercise, heart health, nutrition, body composition, substance use, stress/coping, safety, cancer risk, and osteoporosis risk status before gastric bypass surgery. He went over the first page to make sure I understood how to read the report. The report simply confirmed what I already knew—I needed to manage my diabetes and hypertension, get more sleep, lose a lot of weight, engage in much more aerobic activity, eat fewer high-fat foods, eat breakfast, avoid fast foods and snacking, limit my intake of caffeine, manage my stress, and improve my overall happiness level. My true health age was estimated at 46.7 and the document claimed I could achieve a true body age of 38.2 and add 8.5 years to my life expectancy by changing my health behaviors.

While excited by the prospect of increasing my life expectancy, I was unhappy that I could achieve a body age of only 38. It may be unreasonable to achieve a body age of 20 when one is 44 but why not 35? I asked how often one can have the profile done to track health improvements. The response was every six months. Once I've gotten my weight under control, I will do it again.

Home alone, I spent some time going over the profile. It contained a great deal of useful information. For example, I wasn't aware that obesity increases one's risk of acquiring certain cancers and African Americans are at a lower risk for osteoporosis than white and Asian women. In addition to information about the prevalence of various diseases related to obesity among the American population, the report gives specific details on how to improve one's health. It suggests that with a body mass index of 42.9, weight of 242 pounds, and height of 5 feet 3 inches, I should engage in a fitness program with the goal of achieving a normal body mass of 19–25 and weight of 107–141 pounds. Dynamic weight resistance training and calisthenics at a moderate to high resistance level at a frequency of two days per week are the physical activities that may help me accomplish this. I would need to achieve a target heart rate of 106–133 beats per minute when fitness walking, jogging, bicycling, or swimming at a duration of 20 to 30 minutes per day to start and work my way up to 30 to 60 minutes per day. The Dyna-Bands could be used to do 8 to 10 different weight resistance exercises. The report ended with a chart showing the number of servings I should have each day of grains, vegetables, fruits, dairy, protein, fats, and sweets.

I was provided a packet entitled *Dyna-Band Total Body Toner,* which demonstrated beginner and advanced athletic exercises one can do with the Dyna-Band. You can do exercises for the upper and lower body. Supposedly, anything you can do with free weights or a Nautilus machine you can do with Dyna-Bands. They are extremely convenient. I can watch television in any room of my home and work out with them any time of day.

Even though Mr. Miller seems capable, I will have to find another physical trainer, gym, or be content with the workout equipment in my apartment complex. I prefer to workout in the mornings on days I don't teach. The gym at the hospital, however, is open in the mornings only on Tuesdays and Thursdays, the days I am in the classroom. On Mondays, Wednesdays, and Fridays, the gym is open in the evening only. It is open for a couple of hours on Saturday and not at all on Sunday. In addition, it is a 40-minute round-trip drive through rush-hour traffic to the hospital. I will think seriously about investing in a membership to the YMCA across the street to take advantage of their Iron Abs, Pilates, step aerobics, and swimming classes.

SATURDAY, AUGUST 2, 2003. On *48 Hours* singer Roberta Flack discussed the wonders of a new weight-loss treatment from France called mesotherapy. Her obsession with weight loss began early in her career when a white male television show host commented she would look better if she lost some weight. Even with all of her accomplishments in the music industry, she is most proud of her weight loss. Roberta Flack is a good example of how managing weight for health reasons is becoming secondary to body image concerns for many African Americans.

DISCUSSION QUESTIONS

1. Is weight-loss surgery just another form of plastic surgery? Why or why not?

2. Does the media influence our beliefs about what is aesthetically pleasing and what isn't? Support your position.

3. Should celebrities be obligated to share their illness and health experiences with the public? Why or why not?

4. What role, if any, does religion play in the formation and maintenance of our attitudes toward food?

5. Have you had a personal wellness profile done? If so, what is your "true" body age? Are these profiles scientific and legitimate? Would learning your "true" body age influence you to change your unhealthy behaviors?

SUGGESTED READINGS

Beck, C. S. (2005). Personal stories and public activism: The implications of Michael J. Fox's public health narrative for policy and perspectives. In E. B. Ray (Ed.), *Health communication in practice: A case study approach* (pp. 335–346). Mahwah, NJ: Lawrence Erlbaum Associates.

Casey, M. K., Allen, M., Emmers-Sommer, T., Sahlstein, E., Degooyer, D., Winters, A. M., Wagner, A. E., & Dun, T. (2003). When a celebrity contracts a disease: The example of Earvin "Magic" Johnson's announcement that he was HIV positive. *Journal of Health Communication, 8*(1), 249–256.

Lawrence, R. G. (2004). Framing obesity: The evolution of news discourse on a public health issue. *Harvard International Journal of Press/Politics, 9*(3), 56–75.

10

Weeks Ten through Fifteen Post-Surgery

AUGUST 5–AUGUST 11, 2003. I am adjusting well to my new lifestyle, as evidenced by another successful week with an average of 54 grams of protein consumed per day. Six out of the seven days I managed to eat three meals and two snacks. The snacks were yogurt mixed with Citrucel. During regular meal times, I ate a variety of foods, including hamburger, chicken, pork, beans, broccoli, green beans, pineapple, peaches, and protein bars.

I spent the week vacationing with family in Williamsburg and Virginia Beach, Virginia. On the beach, I sat reading in a full-piece bathing suit with a towel covering my legs hoping no one would notice my large thighs. My body didn't get near the water and I did not stroll up and down the beach. I remained in the same spot for hours until we retuned to the townhouse. As I lay there talking with my sister, I watched my niece, nephew, and brother-in-law enjoy the water together. I felt self-conscious about my weight even though there were many people walking along the beach and laying out who were heavier than me.

My self-consciousness was exacerbated by my niece's apparent fear of taking off the t-shirt that covered her bathing suit even though she said it felt heavy and prevented her from enjoying the water. She would play for a while then approach us and ask "Should I take my shirt off?" over and over again. The question and her body consciousness surprised me and caught me off guard. Generally, my teenage niece is a self-assured, confident, and outgoing person. Each time she posed the question, I became more and more aware of how our American obsession with body image was impacting us both.

I did not want to make her uncomfortable and overly body conscious. I told her to do what was most comfortable for her. At the same time, I was aware that others were staring at her. This made me sad, angry, and ashamed for them and for myself because I didn't think she should take off her t-shirt and subject her overweight body to ridicule and mean-spirited talk. Did I think she should be embarrassed, or was I more concerned about my own embarrassment? I tried to think about other things and told myself that how my family members looked and acted did not reflect on me. What bull we tell ourselves! For most of the day she kept the t-shirt on and I felt more at ease.

Overall, vacationing with my sister and her family was wonderful. I was able to exercise on the workout equipment at the complex and eat out and bring the leftovers back to use in other meals. I learned that I can adapt to different situations and environments and still eat properly. During our time together I tried to influence my family by making smoothies with yogurt and a variety of fruits. They drank them to make me happy although I know they didn't particularly care for them. That's okay. It feels good to know that they made every attempt to spare my feelings. Nevertheless, I am perplexed. Even though I averaged 50 minutes of intense exercise for five out of seven days this week, and got in a reasonable amount of exercise through shopping at all of the outlet malls in the area, I did not lose a pound. On a positive note, at least I did not gain any weight, either.

AUGUST 12–AUGUST 18, 2003. I got in 58 grams of protein per day and worked out four out of seven days this week for an average of 60 minutes! My goal is to exercise for an hour every day that I work out from this point onward and work my way into exercising a minimum of five days a week. At work everyone seems to be dieting and sharing healthy eating tips. My menu of appropriate foods remains the same and I am taking the same medications and vitamins.

News reports today announced the death of Idi Amin due to kidney disease and failure. This morbidly obese dictator and mass murderer of hundreds of Africans exemplifies everything I dislike about living an affluent lifestyle—the tendency toward excess. If anyone deserved to suffer and die as a result of the complications of obesity, it was Idi Amin, not my mother. God, why did my mother have to suffer?

AUGUST 19–AUGUST 25, 2003. I averaged 53 minutes of exercise per day and 58 grams of protein, eating many of the same foods and taking the same medications and vitamins. I did branch out and included yellow squash, zucchini, cabbage, and honeydew melon in my diet. On the 20th, I met with my nutritionist's assistant to have my weight loss documented. Amy weighed me in at 202.7 (2 lbs less than my home scale) and raved that I had lost 20 pounds in one month. When she asked what I thought was the key factor in losing the weight, I said intense exercise—not simply strolling through the neighborhood, but intense workouts on the treadmill and stationary bike and the incorporation of Dyna-Bands for resistance training.

Amy handed me a form entitled "10 Weeks Post Op." I quickly scanned it and asked her how it differed from the previous meal form I received. She could not tell me. The first addition I saw was a small salad with low fat dressing. The sheet reminded me to avoid trouble foods such as alcohol, sweets, and fatty foods. I read: "Think of those foods as your enemy . . . and think of how you feel right now . . . maybe 40 or more pounds less than you were before surgery . . . are those foods worth going back to the old you?" I thought, *hell no!* I have lost nearly 50 pounds and I don't want to gain a single ounce back! I continued reading: "Water—exercise—measure—eat—healthy—be healthy—be happy with yourself!" I like that! Yes, it feels good to know that you can do what you need to do to get healthier. I like what I do for me!

The paper included a list of many of the technical names for sugar and encouraged food label reading and the avoidance of foods with more than 14 grams of sugar per serving. I have already made it a habit to avoid foods that have more than 12 grams per serving. Richard Simmons' "Project Me Passport" was included in the handout. This exercise guru was in town last month and many of my fellow support group members worked out with him. His "passport" simply suggests that the overweight person own up to her responsibility in her weight problem and simply do what is necessary to change—"eat healthy, exercise, and stay motivated." What I found most interesting was the announcement for the 2003 National Weight Loss Surgery Convention scheduled for the last week in August in Nashville, Tennessee. I couldn't believe that they actually have conventions for people who have had weight-loss surgery! Wow! I wonder what they are like but will probably never know because I just can't see myself attending one.

There was a recipe for popcorn garlic shrimp and a list of high-protein snacks that I wasn't aware of including Lean Protein Bites, Soy Protein Chips, and UTurn Bars, all of which could be purchased at GNC or CVS. Sixteen ounces of Diet Snapple with 4 grams of sugar and 20 calories was listed as a sugar-free drink that one could have one week post-op. The paper also announced that our surgeon, Dr. Bozeman, was now performing a new lap-band procedure that was less invasive and drastic than the surgery I had. I left the office refreshed and looked forward to trying the new items listed.

MONDAY, AUGUST 25. I ran into one of my former students on campus. Jennifer has serious medical problems and has had to make numerous changes in her lifestyle, particularly about diet. We've had numerous conversations in the past and I knew how seriously she took the topic of health care. Although young, she has an intellect that one can only acquire through personal sustained experience. She actually mistook me for a student, which was flattering, and commented, "You look wonderful and less stressed." We went into my office and talked for a while openly sharing our surgery, lifestyle, and diet experiences. Jennifer was excited and happy for me, and I was happy to hear that her health was gradually improving to the point that she could attend classes full time. She asked if she could share my story with another of my former students who was having problems with obesity. Permission was granted and I asked her to encourage the student to come speak with me personally.

Later that evening I spoke with one of my best friends, Kai, on the phone. Kai, who lives in Texas, told me that another of our friends, T, who lives in Ohio, was considering weight-loss surgery. Apparently, T's mother was really pressing the issue. Kai was concerned that weight-loss surgery wasn't the appropriate solution for T because of her other health problems, especially her tendency to bleed heavily each month, which resulted in severe anemia and the need for transfusions on a regular basis. She was concerned also that T would not be able to make and sustain the necessary lifestyle changes. T was primarily concerned that she might die during surgery because one of her acquaintances had a sister who died on the operating table. I explained to Kai that death was rare although a possibility with this type of surgery, and even with the most minor of surgeries one must seriously consider death as a risk.

The announcer on *Entertainment Tonight* said there are rumors that one of the stars of *The View*, Star Jones, is considering weight-loss surgery and if she has the surgery Barbara Walters would be documenting her progress. Neither would confirm nor deny the rumors.

AUGUST 26–SEPTEMBER 1, 2003. My friend Rana is planning to run in a marathon at Virginia Beach during the Labor Day weekend. She runs to raise money for the Kentucky Lymphoma and Leukemia Society. I'm not a runner, although I do my part by sending her a check for the cause. She is an extraordinarily charitable person and is blessed in many ways because of it. In her e-mail she asked how my first day of class went. My response focused on the state of shock that many of my former students were experiencing at my weight loss. I am really amazed at how drastic weight loss can leave normally verbose individuals totally speechless. They didn't know how to react to me. One student did find his voice and managed to utter while shaking his head from side to side in apparent disbelief, "What have you been doing? Amazing! Impressive! It is really amazing! I commend you!" I thanked him for noticing and walked away.

Throughout the work week, other students in my classes found their tongues and commented on my weight loss. One pointed her finger at me, shook her head from side to side for emphases, and stated empathetically, "You—look—GOOD!" Even one of my co-workers who had seen me all summer but had not commented finally acknowledged the change with, "You really look nice. I meant to say something last week. I can tell you made some changes in your hair, clothes, and—lost weight. You really look good!" The acknowledgements were appreciated. Although, as the saying goes, *one day up, and the next one, down.*

TUESDAY, SEPTEMBER 2, 2003. When I came in to work I turned on the radio to listen to a morning talk show as I prepared for my classes. The hosts, one white female and one white male, were discussing Randy Jackson, one of the judges of the popular television program *American Idol*. Randy had laparoscopic gastric bypass surgery and had begun to show weight loss. The conversation was extremely negative with the hosts suggesting that such behavior was stupid and on a par with having plastic surgery. Randy Jackson was accused of "getting on the Carnie Wilson/Al Roker bandwagon." The male host laughingly commented, "It's like supergluing your nostrils shut to manage a cocaine problem."

I was outraged! Livid! How could any intelligent human being equate dealing with a weight problem with a cocaine addiction? I wanted to wring those fools' necks! Clearly, many people do not understand what weight-loss surgery is all about. They don't understand that it is not a simple fix in which one's weight problem is solved in the matter of an hour. *It is a lifelong lifestyle change!* And, it *ain't* easy! Do talk show hosts understand the impact of their words? What harm might have one of these jerks done to someone who may seriously be considering this *legal,* medical option? Calm down.

When I returned from class, the secretary asked me how my co-workers were reacting to my weight loss. I mentioned that not all of them had commented on it and a few were acting as if nothing had happened, even though I didn't see how one could ignore a co-worker losing more than 50 pounds. She suggested they had all noticed but that a few might be jealous and find it difficult to be supportive of me when they were dealing with their own weight issues. One in particular had a baby nearly two years before and had not lost the weight gained through pregnancy.

True, others may be dealing with their own weight issues. But, who better to talk and commiserate with than me? I think it is thoughtless and rude to not acknowledge someone else's success. One thing I do know—when one of them loses weight, I will acknowledge it. Hey, no hard feelings. Life is much too short!

DISCUSSION QUESTIONS

1. Have you ever been embarrassed by a family member's weight? Why? When? Does the weight of your family members reflect on who you are as a person? Why or why not?

2. What is a healthy diet? Where do you get the best information on healthy eating? When you receive contradictory messages, how do you decide who to believe?

3. What do you do to assist our institutions in solving health problems? Do we as citizens have a responsibility to support research aimed at improving health in the population?

SUGGESTED READINGS

Bowen, D. J., Singal, R., Eng, E., Crystal, S., & Burke, W. (2003). Jewish identity and intentions to obtain breast cancer screening. *Cultural Diversity and Ethnic Minority Psychology*, *9*(1), 78–87.

Kreps, G. L. (2005). Narrowing the digital divide to overcome disparities in care. In E. B. Ray (Ed.), *Health communication in practice: A case study approach* (pp. 357–364). Mahwah, NJ: Lawrence Erlbaum Associates.

11

A New Life in a New City

When I started my weight loss journey, I weighed 248 pounds, had a 45-inch waist, 52-inch hips, and 46-inch breast size with a DD cup. By May 2004, I had lost more than 100 pounds and had been able to maintain the weight loss through regular exercise and healthy eating. My waist is 26 inches, hips 38 inches, breasts 36 inches and I can barely fill a B cup. Although I have yet to reach my goal weight of 140 pounds or less, I feel healthier than I have ever felt as an adult.

Recently I found a letter from November 1998 in which my doctor, Dr. Shultz, stated, "Your C-peptide was elevated at 3 nanograms per milliliter indicating definite insulin resistance indicative of obesity and probably a pre-diabetic state. Hopefully, a low carbohydrate diet and a regular aerobics exercise program will help you control your weight and reduce the likelihood of diabetes for the future." I reflected on how this letter, at the time, meant little to me. My concern was on finding a new doctor since he was retiring, and I felt I had plenty of time to address my weight issue since the blood test suggested everything else was normal. If I had taken his diagnosis and suggestions seriously in addition to having the knowledge I have now, I would have acted sooner. Today, I do not take anything lightly when it comes to my health.

In July 2004, I moved to Florida to begin teaching at the University of Miami. Before I left North Carolina, I signed forms for all of my doctors to release information to whatever new doctors I found in Florida. In addition, I packed all my health records and the names and addresses of all of my former doctors for easy reference. Many of my new co-workers recommended their doctors to me and I was able to find a doctor of internal medicine to fit my needs. However I did have to change insurance companies twice in less than two years.

In Miami, I am not a fat girl. None of my co-workers knew me as a fat girl and the fact that they do not know I am a reformed fat girl has given me a new sense of freedom. I am reminded every day, however, that I had gastric bypass surgery. My food portions remain small because my stomach will not allow me to eat normal "American" portions. My taste for various foods changes constantly. For example, before the surgery, I ate salads with lettuce and tomato regularly. Now the mere sight or smell of fresh lettuce and tomatoes makes me nauseated. I rarely eat eggs, and a French fry will send me running to the bathroom immediately. I have to taste-test everything I did not personally cook, and I rarely eat out. When I do, it is purely for social reasons, and when I am not careful in choosing the right foods, I get sick. Nevertheless, I do not regret my decision to have gastric bypass surgery.

Within months of my arrival in Florida, my Aunt Annie passed away from complications of diabetes and hypertension. Luther Vandross finally succumbed to his complications of diabetes in July 2005, and on the morning of February 17, 2006, my second mom, Mac, died of pancreatic cancer. Between February and April of 2006, my hypertensive twin sister had a stroke and was diagnosed with breast cancer. She is currently undergoing chemotherapy and radiation treatments. On June 16, 2006, I learned the father of my childhood friend Chuck was hospitalized. His father, who had lived with diabetes for most of his adult life, was now receiving dialysis several days a week.

I see poor health and death around me everywhere, and I am obsessed with my health primarily because many of my days are filled now with handling the physical costs of my decision to have weight-loss surgery. In early November of 2005, I had a physical, mammogram, and a series of blood tests to determine my health status after experiencing pain deep in the bones of my arms. My urine, electrolytes, potassium, kidney functioning, glucose, calcium, folate, vitamin B, iron, magnesium, and cholesterol levels were all normal. The X-ray of my upper body indicated nothing. However, the blood test determined I was menopausal, and a radiologist demanded additional views of my right breast after viewing the results of my mammogram.

At the end of November 2005, I learned I had a vitamin D deficiency and parathyroidism. I was instructed to take 800 international units of vitamin D daily. Even though sun exposure is perhaps the most important source of vitamin D and abundant in the Sunshine State, my body is unable to absorb enough vitamin D through my digestive track. The surgical removal and manipulation of part of my stomach and intestines has impaired my digestion and ability to absorb many nutrients. Aging also leads to an increased risk of developing this deficiency because the kidney becomes less able to convert vitamin D to its active hormone form. Additionally, people with darker skin have a more difficult time absorbing vitamin D from sunlight, especially if they have low rates of casual sunlight exposure. As a result, African American women are at a greater risk of vitamin D deficiency than white women.

In early March of 2006, I was informed that my bone density test indicated "osteoperia," low bone mass. Osteoporosis, a disease characterized by fragile bones and an increase in bone fractures, is most often associated with inadequate calcium intake and a vitamin D deficiency. My blood tests reported my calcium, parathyroid hormone, and phosphorous levels were normal but my vitamin D level was still low. I was instructed to increase the amount of vitamin D that I was taking twice daily. The constant breakdown and rebuilding of bone due to menopause, in addition to my vitamin D deficiency, osteoporosis, and malabsorption due to gastric bypass surgery explained my nagging bone pain and muscle weakness. To manage this problem, I take 2000 international units of vitamin D a day and work out with weights a minimum of three times a week. Should I be angry because of these events? Maybe, but I am not. That consent form I signed warned me of these possible consequences of gastric bypass surgery.

Life goes on and as human beings we adapt. In January 2006, there was a problem with my mammographic findings and an area of my breast needed further evaluation. I had the mammogram films for the 3 previous years sent from the Charlotte Radiology Breast Center so the Miami radiologist could make comparisons for an optimal evaluation. In each of these previous mammograms there was no indication of breast cancer. Thankfully, my Miami radiologist determined my mammogram "showed a stable appearance" in comparison with the three previous ones. My ultrasound was normal. Nevertheless, my doctors suggested I have a mammogram every 6 months to watch for changes in my right breast.

Today I find I can eat larger portions of food. However, I cannot eat the large super-sized portions that the average American eats. Sometimes I feel twinges of hunger when I go without eating for three to four hours; and at other times I have to fight the urge to eat that which is satisfying but unhealthy. The urge has won out more times than I care to admit.

In addition, my desire to exercise wanes rather than increases. I can exercise every day for up to two hours for weeks and then not exercise at all for an entire week. Consequently, maintaining my weight loss has become a daily challenge. I have gained weight and lost it again. Nevertheless, my commitment to lead a healthy lifestyle remains strong. To get back on course and jolt me back into action, all I have to do is look at a picture of my mother and step on the bathroom scale.

DISCUSSIONS QUESTIONS

1. In considering the entire narrative, how would you characterize Dr. Drummond's overall attitude toward health? What specific

beliefs or values can you identity? Did you see any inconsistencies between attitudes expressed and behaviors enacted? What persuasion theories best explain Dr. Drummond's overall attitudes and behavior?

2. What are some of the common euphemisms we use when people die? Why do we feel uncomfortable talking about death? What cultural differences exist in dealing with death?

THEORIES TO CONTEXTUALIZE DISCUSSION

Narrative Theory suggests storytelling is intrinsic to human nature. Some individuals tell better stories than others. We judge the coherence and fidelity of stories to assess narrative logic. Ultimately, those stories that are most compelling and persuasive become the basis for social action. To learn more about this approach, read the works of W. R. Fisher:

Fisher, W. R. (1987). *Human communication as narration: Toward a philosophy of reason, value, and action.* Columbia, SC: University of South Carolina Press.

Fisher, W. R. (1995). Narration, knowledge and the possibility of wisdom. In R. F. Goodman & W. R. Fisher (Eds.), *Rethinking knowledge* (pp. 169–192). Albany, NY: SUNY Press.

The Theory of Reasoned Action is based on the assumption that we consciously and deliberately make decisions. Each decision made is based primarily on two considerations: (1) how strongly we believe engaging in a specific behavior will lead to positive outcomes for us, and (2) an evaluation of what the social consequences will be for engaging in the behavior. For a strong grounding in this theory, read:

Ajzen, I., & Fishbein, M. (1980). *Understanding attitudes and predicting behavior.* Englewood Cliffs, NJ: Prentice-Hall.

The Elaboration Likelihood Model assumes there are two major ways persuasion occurs. Either an individual will carefully scrutinize a message and be influenced by the strength of the arguments made, or one will fail to think about message content and be persuaded by things peripheral to the message such as the speaker's physical attractiveness. For more about this model, go straight to the source:

Petty, R. E., & Cacioppo, J. T. (1986). *Communication and persuasion: Central and peripheral routes to attitude change.* New York: Springer-Verlag.

The Communication Theory of Identity and its extension, **Cultural Contracts Theory,** both suggest that identities are multidimensional and negotiated with personal, enacted, relational, and communal frames of reference that help us understand our communicative encounters. Our identities are negotiated via cultural contracts throughout the term of our relationships. The best resource for learning more about these theories is:

Hecht, M. L., Jackson, R. L., & Ribeau, S. A. (2003). *African American communication: Exploring identity and culture* (2nd ed). Mahwah, NJ: Lawrence Erlbaum Associates.

Index